Reiki

Healing for

Beginners

How to Improve Your Health by Channeling and
Strengthening the Chakra Energy

(How to Use Crystals & Chakras to Improve
Health, Body & Life and to Increase and Balance
Your Energy)

Lawrence Brennan

Published by Rob Miles

Lawrence Brennan

Reiki Healing for Beginners: How to Improve Your Health by Channeling and Strengthening the Chakra Energy (How to Use Crystals & Chakras to Improve Health, Body & Life and to Increase and Balance Your Energy)

ISBN 978-1-989990-30-8

Legal & Disclaimer

The information contained in this book is not designed to replace or take the place of any form of medicine or professional medical advice. The information in this book has been provided for educational and entertainment purposes only.

The information contained in this book has been compiled from sources deemed reliable, and it is accurate to the best of the Author's knowledge; however, the Author cannot guarantee its accuracy and validity and cannot be held liable for any errors or omissions. Changes are periodically made to this book. You must consult your doctor or get professional medical advice before using any of the suggested remedies, techniques, or information in this book.

Upon using the information contained in this book, you agree to hold harmless the Author from and against any damages, costs, and expenses, including any legal fees potentially resulting from the application of any of the information provided by this guide. This disclaimer applies to any damages or injury caused by the use and application, whether directly or indirectly, of any advice or information presented, whether for breach of contract, tort, negligence, personal injury, criminal intent, or under any other cause of action.

You agree to accept all risks of using the information presented inside this book. You need to consult a professional medical practitioner in order to ensure you are both able and healthy enough to participate in this program.

Table of Contents

Introduction

The following chapters in this book are meant to help beginners learn exactly what Reiki is and how they can incorporate it into their everyday life. Some of you may have heard the term Reiki before, or have a bit of knowledge about what exactly it is. Others may never have heard of it, and simply picked this book up out of curiosity. Regardless of your background, this book is full of useful information for everyone and will help prepare you for either learning Reiki or for going to your very first session.

Energy healing is a powerful tool that can help anyone who is suffering mentally, emotionally, spiritually, or even physically. It has been used for centuries to treat a wide variety of different illnesses and ailments and continues to be used to this very day. Reiki healers are trained in these techniques, and they have learned how to take their internal energy and transfer it into someone else in order to assist them. Internal energy exists within all of us, but very few of us know how to tap into it and unleash its powers. That is why Reiki is so important, as it teaches us how to use that which already exists but is often ignored.

From the individual chakras all the way to your main aura, Reiki healing taps into all of your energy sources and works to align and balance them so that you are the best version of yourself possible. You don't need to suffer from sickness, stress, anxiety, or depression, and instead can use this natural method to free yourself from that suffering.

In order to get the most out of this book, it is important that you go into it with an open mind. Each chapter will explore a variety of different concepts, and you will come across terms and ideas that you are unfamiliar with. Our natural human reaction, when presented with something different, is to shy away, but by embracing this information and welcoming it with open arms, you can learn an entirely new way of living.

Give yourself the gift of health, and learn why Reiki is such a powerful way of transforming who you are. Even if you are physically healthy, the day to day stress that we all experience can build up and create blocks within our energy systems. Reiki assists us in removing those blocks, eliminating our stress, and making us better equipped at handling whatever life throws our way. From feeling stronger and more confident, to be able to better communicate with friends and loved ones, Reiki impacts us on a multitude of levels and is absolutely worth learning more about.

There are plenty of books on this subject on the market, thanks again for choosing this one! Every effort was made to ensure it is full of as much useful information as possible. Please enjoy!

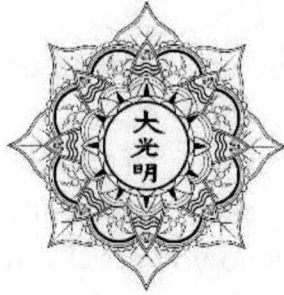

Chapter 1: Understand Reiki And Its Benefits

The ancient Japanese way of healing someone through massaging their main parts such as shoulder, head, hands and feet is the most relaxing one ever. The spiritual practice is not related to the religion at all but you can relieve your stress through the Reiki sessions where your body and mind releases any tension it has. You will feel a balance between the mind and body when you go through the Reiki sessions. If you want a mental clarity and some peace in your brain then you have to get the Reiki sessions once in a life and you will be able to feel the difference. Reiki has healed a lot of patients who fall into depression or sadness. It works as the best psychologist practices around the world because of its healing power.

You can improve your life through Reiki sessions so here are some of the benefits which you get once you attend the 30 minutes session of Reiki.

It reduces the stress and anxiety from your body with keeping it relaxed all the time. The nature body triggers the immune system to stay strong and you will be able to sleep deep. When you wake up, you will feel how much better it is with the improved health physically and mentally.

Helps you maintain the inner peace and harmony with growing the spiritual feeling inside you.

It helps you to balance the emotions and mind at the same time. If you are someone who tends to stay annoyed at most of the things and feels irritated on little things, then it can surely calm you down. Tension causes the change in the moods which is why it is important to attend the sessions. It can elevate the mood and even get you rid of frustration and anger. It can work best to fix your relationships because the more relaxed you will be, you will be able to pay attention to your relationships and make it stronger.

You will be able to love without any tension and it can open up your brain to make your relationships sustain and grown. You will see an increase in the empathy and it allows you to connect to the people who are around you by keeping you calm.

There will be no sorrow in your brain after attending the Reiki session. It cleans the emotions by draining and giving you a new perspective towards life which you will surely love.

It helps you get rid of the diseases such as menopausal symptoms, insomnia, asthma, fatigue, arthritis, migraine and much more. If you have any long term illness, you will be able to get over it without any chaos. You do not have to be worried about it once you go through the session.

It helps you to heal immediate problems as well such as if you are going through a relationship breakup, it helps you get over the negative emotions and helps to maintain the balance to come back to the regular life.

There are no restrictions for Reiki sessions. Anyone can attend it such as the babies, children and adults. There are no harms of Reiki and it definitely changes your lifestyle to a better mode than before. You can also have the consultation sessions while having Reiki which helps you get over the stress in your brain. When you have stressed yourself, your entire body reacts to it and leaves its effects such as it can leave you a headache and you will not be able to get over it unless the problem is solved. With Reiki, you will be able to manage the daily life stress easily and keep the moods normal as well.

Chapter 2: Advantages Of Using Reiki As A System For Healing And Self-Healing

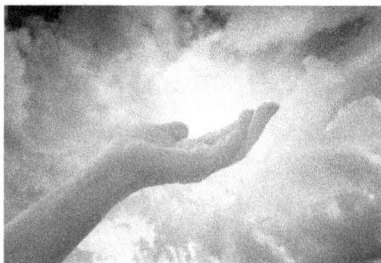

There are many bodywork styles that can work well with the physical, energetic, and emotional bodies. Massage therapy, acupuncture, chiropractic adjustments, and reflexology are all well known and have amazing benefits. Reiki is a more unique style of bodywork because it is highly intuitive and doesn't require extensive knowledge of anatomy. With Reiki, you don't intend to target specific parts of the body, Reiki energy goes where it is most needed.

However, there are benefits to knowing the basics of human anatomy and how it relates to different symptoms. Even if you only plan on using Reiki on yourself, understanding the different relationships between key systems in the body, you'll better be able to trace the source of your symptoms.

All symptoms that present in the body, whether it is physical pain, illness, injury, or disease, stem from an energetic imbalance in the body which creates dis-ease. Dis-ease opens the doors and windows for the body to be incapable of functioning at its optimal health and wellness levels. When the body can't function at those levels it begins to experience problems in the body systems which then lead to pain, illness, injury, and disease.

Symptoms of dis-ease can also manifest in an emotional or spiritual way. Many mental health conditions can be a result of dis-ease. As can the manifestation of trauma and anxiety disorders. Obsessive compulsive disorder, attention deficit disorder, nightmares, they can also be results of imbalance and dis-ease in the body.

Using Reiki to treat symptoms of dis-ease will eventually lead back to the root cause. In many cases, knowing the root cause of the dis-ease is only half the battle. Once you've identified a cause within yourself, you may need to take extra steps to change your lifestyle in order to prevent the dis-ease from coming back. Healing comes from within, which is why self-healing is the most effective path towards a more positive, empowered lifestyle.

Again, this is why Reiki is so amazing, because you can use it to heal yourself. During a self-treatment session, you can discover the root cause of your symptoms through the intuitive experiences you have when treating yourself. If you receive Reiki sessions from other practitioners, you may not get the same intuitive information.

11

Your Reiki Practitioner will probably pickup on certain imbalances in you through visions and sensations, but they won't be able to interpret what those visions and sensations mean to you. You will have to discover the meanings for yourself and what you can change in your life to prevent the dis-ease from returning.

When performing Reiki sessions on others, your intuition might guide you to sources of their dis-ease. However, since healing comes from within, you can only guide them in the right direction. You can never interpret what something means to someone else for them. Nor can you tell them the best way to resolve whatever conflicts they are experiencing. This is why self-healing is so important.

Knowing enough basic anatomy on the energetic, physical, and emotional level you can better understand what you feel and what the sources of your own dis-ease is.

Chakras

The chakra system is comprised of seven main chakras that sit along the spine. There are additional sub chakras throughout the body with as many as up to one hundred and fourteen.

Chakra translated from Sanskrit means disk or wheel. Chakras are spinning energetic pools that connect the physical body, the energetic body, and the emotional body. They are the convergence point of the three bodies coming together. They are the centers of energy in the body, with a swirling energy that rotates in both a clockwise and counterclockwise directions.

The chakras are cone shaped. The apex of the cone is right on the spine and then the cone extends outwards in both the front and the back of the body. The two exceptions are the crown chakra which expands up from the top of the head and the root chakra which expands down towards the feet out the tail of the spine.

The seven main chakras are the crown chakra at the top of the head. The third eye chakra at the crown and occiput. The throat chakra at the base of the throat and the top of the shoulder blades. The heart chakra at the center of the sternum and between the shoulder blades on the back. The solar plexus chakra an inch or two above the naval and above the sacrum. The sacral chakra an in or two below the naval and at the sacrum. The root chakra is at the base of the spine.

Each chakra resonates with a body cavity, organs, and organ systems. These chakras also align with emotional and energetic components of the body, mind, and spirit. This is how energetic imbalances and dis-ease can then contribute to manifestations of illness, disease, injury, and emotional conditions and disorders. Since the chakras are so connected to different layers of the body, they can be a source of imbalance that presents moderate to severe symptoms.

Reiki is a balancing healing modality. It resonates well with the chakras and helps to realign their energies, thus resulting in fewer symptoms and a healthier life. How Reiki can be used with and benefit the chakras is going to be elaborated on in future chapters. Another book in this series Chakras Healing for Beginners is another source of how the chakras and Reiki energy work together.

Chakras are a well-known part of the energetic anatomy and the physical anatomy. There are plenty of ways to balance and heal the chakras. One of the benefits of Reiki is that Reiki can be sent over time and space. It can be used to heal deeply rooted past traumas that may have been repressed, or even forgotten about. These traumas never fully go away, but might become overshadowed by the manifestation of more prevalent or current symptoms. Imbalances that go unaddressed can end up in a much different place than where they started.

Aura

The aura is another commonly known energetic system that is part of the body. Think of your aura like a personal bubble. The concept of the personal bubble derives from the aura. The aura is an electromagnetic energy frequency that is projected by your individual energetic vibration.

The aura can be expanded out away from the body or retracted to be closer to the body. The health of your aura is going to contribute to your physical, mental, and emotional health as well. Your aura is in a sense, a shield for you and energies around you. It can protect you from unwanted energies, but if it is unhealthy or imbalanced this protection is greatly diminished.

The aura is also a tool for you to attract people and situations in your life that resonate with your personal energy. Energies attract and repel each other. If your aura is raised to the energetic frequency that you most strongly align with, then other people, jobs, and life situations that are going to compliment you and your personal power.

Around your body, the aura exists in seven layers. Each layer corresponds to one of the seven main chakras. The first layer of the aura is about 1-2 inches from the body and resonates with the root chakra. The second auric layer is roughly 3-4 inches from the body and correlates to the sacral chakra. The third layer of the aura sits 5-6 inches from the body and it is related to the solar plexus chakra. The fourth auric layer is between 7-8 inches from the body and it resonates with the heart chakra.

The fifth layer of the aura is the pastel color layer. It relates to the throat chakra and is about 9-10 inches from the body. This is the colored layer that can be seen as a reflection of your personal energetic vibration. The sixth layer of the aura resonates with the third eye chakra and rests between 11 and 12 inches from the body. It is a silver light layer that is a shield for you against unwanted and negative energies. The seventh aura later is about 13-14 inches from the body and correlates to the crown chakra. The seventh layer is comprised of beads. These beads can become cracked or damaged over time due to exposure to all the energies in the world. The beads wear down over time and need to be refreshed.

Reiki energy healing is a wonderful form of energy that helps balance the aura. It realigns the layers with the chakras and rejuvenates your personal protective bubble.

Lymphatic System

The lymphatic system is one of the main components of the immune system. Comprised of lymphatic vessels, lymphatic ducts and lymph nodes. Lymph is a fluid that runs through the lymphatic vessels and helps remove waste from the body, organs, and organ systems.

The thoracic duct in the chest is the main vessel of the lymphatic system. Unlike the circulatory system that has the heart to pump blood through your veins, the lymphatic system requires bodily movement to keep lymph flowing properly.

This is one reason that exercise and movement is so important to the health of the body. Without it, lymph doesn't flow properly. This leads to blockages in the system. It also leads to improper cleaning of the body and deteriorates the functionality of the immune system.

Overtime this leads to many issues in the body on a physical, mental, and spiritual level. It can be hard to trace these blocks back to the lymphatic system, especially because they are physical blocks, not necessarily energetic blocks. An energetic imbalance in one of the chakras can lead to a lack of motivation or energy which results in a lack of movement and exercise, thus becoming an issue with the lymphatic system.

Reiki is a subtle energy. It is noninvasive. Yet it stimulates the energetic currents in the body, like the nervous system electrical impulses. It can balance the chakras that link to motivation and energy, which can provide you with the personal power to begin moving and exercising, even if it is just for a twenty minute walk every day.

The lymphatic system is a part of the physical anatomy, but it has strong ties to the energetic anatomy. Since it is a part of the immune system and without proper energetic balance, the immune system weakens, the two together are closely entwined. This correlation is another reason that Reiki energy is such a powerful healing tool for the lymphatic system.

The thoracic duct of the lymphatic system closely resonates with the heart chakra and can be stimulated by the static hand positions of a Reiki treatment placed over the heart chakra. When combined with other healing methods such as crystals, this can enhance the focus of Reiki energy specifically on the heart chakra or the thoracic duct. Even though Reiki is intuitive by nature, it can be focused with the implementation of other healing methods like crystals.

Muscular System

Muscles in the body are a source of structure, movement, and strength. Muscles move the bones and joints which move the limbs. Muscles move the mouth to assist with speech and facial expressions.

Movement is a source of energy in the body. If the muscles are imbalanced, then this can result in a lack of movement and a lack of energy flow in the body. The muscular system is controlled by electrical impulses from the nervous system. Electricity is another form of energetic current in the body.

Muscles, ligaments, and tendons are all part of the muscular system. Fascia connective tissue is part of the muscular system.

The muscular system can also become a major source of pain and discomfort in the body. Muscular pain is some of the hardest to diagnose unless there is a torn or ripped tendon, ligament or muscle. There are over six hundred muscles in the human body. Determining what exact muscle is the source of pain and then what is causing that pain can become quite difficult. MRI's and X-rays only do so much when looking at the muscular system.

When it comes to connective tissue like fascia, a lot of the information on fascia is still new and surfacing in the medical community. Conditions such as plantar fasciitis have been somewhat controversial in the past.

The muscles have such a connection with different energetic currents in the body, it is no wonder that Reiki energy healing can balance and benefit the muscles so profoundly. Reiki interacts with the kinetic energy, potential energy, and the electrical energy of the muscles. When there is an energetic imbalance this means that there can be an overactivity in energy or a block somewhere in the system.

Fortunately, with Reiki, you do not need to know if there is a block or an overactivity in order for Reiki to heal the imbalance. Different symptoms might present for a block as for overactive energy. With Reiki, you don't need to know the nature of the imbalance because Reiki intuitively goes where it is needed and works on the energetic imbalances. It might take several sessions for you to experience relief or notice changes in the imbalances. Sometimes, the results are so subtle, you might not notice them right away.

With the muscular system, imbalances often lead to pain and injury, so the results of Reiki healing may be more noticeable.

Endocrine Systems

When it comes to functionality of the body, the endocrine system is one of the most important systems. The endocrine system includes glands and controls the production and excretion of hormones and enzymes. Hormones control homeostasis in the body. Hormones assist with sexuality, fertility, and even emotional responses. Enzymes assist with digestion and other functions in the body.

The thyroid gland, adrenal glands, ovaries, salivary glands, testis, pituitary glands, and all the other glands in the body are a part of the endocrine system. These glands produce and excrete the hormones and enzymes that contribute to the balance in your body.

Anyone who has had a hormone disorder, or a problem with their thyroid gland, or even severe mood swings during menstruation have had experiences with severe hormonal imbalances.

The chakras correlate with specific glands and their hormones. This means that an energetic imbalance in the chakras can lead to a gland or hormone disorder or disease. Reiki energy balances those chakras and keeps the endocrine system balanced, producing hormones and enzymes appropriately.

The body can be thrown completely out of functioning parameters if the endocrine system isn't working. The immune system can fail, fertility problems can arise, lack of sexual interest or libido, and emotional problems can result. Other issues such as the inability to make decisions and not being able to think rationally are also impacted by the endocrine system.

It is important to keep the endocrine system producing and secreting hormones and enzymes within balance. Reiki energy healing can correct imbalances and bring the endocrine system back into alignment leading to a healthy body, mind, and spirit.

Chapter 3: Magic Money Box

Money is an integral part of human life. We need money to survive. Without money, we cannot even purchase anything to survive. We would end up being a poor homeless person. Apart from essential use of money, we need money to follow our passions and fulfill our dreams and goals. Below is a small way you can attract more money to fulfill your wishes and goals.

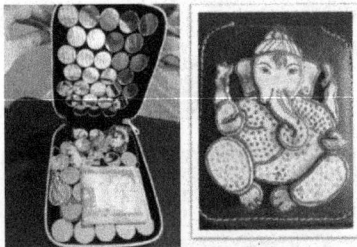

The inside and outside of my magic money box.
Lord Ganesha wooden cutout on top.
First and foremost thing to do is to cleanse your surroundings. Let go of

"access baggage". De-clutter your work space and home. Invoke symbols and Archangels to cleanse and purify your surroundings. Burn sage and incense sticks for purification. If possible, put this magic money box in southeast corner of your house or workplace.

To make a Magic Money Box-

1. Take a box that attracts you. It could be anything, a shoebox, small carton or a jewelry box of any size, any shape. Take time to decorate it. Put all your heart in decorating the magic box. Imagine your financial goals manifesting while you decorate your magic money box. You can use anything to decorate, wrapping paper, stones, shells, colors, glitters, whatever attracts you.

2. Take mirrors of the size that can fit in the box. You need minimum two mirrors. Maximum no limit. When the number of mirrors in all the sides of the box are added they should be even. Mirrors can be

placed on 2, 4 or 6 sides of the box facing each other in parallel.

3. Stick the mirror on the inside base of the box and on inside top of the box (Lid). If you want to add more mirrors, stick on sides too. Keep in mind that the number of mirrors has to be even numbers when added in total.

4. Take a piece of paper (green if possible), make intention slips based on finance, abundance or prosperity, stating your wishes clearly. You can also put money-affirmations. Draw symbols that you are attuned to on the back side of paper.

5. Add the things that project money in the box. Citrine, Aventurine, Cash, Jewelry etc. Do not use fake jewelry as it does not represent real money.

6. Take a candle (green if possible) and lit it. The reason for the paper and candle being green is simply because the color green attracts and symbolizes money. Place your ready magic box beside the

candle. Read out your intentions aloud or in mind. Visualize your wishes being manifested. Call upon your angels and request them to keep your money box charged and flowing with fortune. Blow the candle and thank the Angels and the Universe.

7. Give healing to the magic money box daily. Burn sage or incense stick around the area where you keep the box, so as to keep the area pure and devoid of negative vibes.

8. Once your wish is manifested, invoke symbols and angels. Thank symbols and angels and burn the slip.

Personally, I placed one affirmation only. "I love money. Money loves me and comes to me easily." Within one month of making the box, we bought two laptops (My husband was against buying even one new laptop earlier). After another month I started festive-crafting business. Next, hubby bought few gold jewelry for me and daughter. I thank my magic money box daily. I am saving more money than before.

My only advice to whoever tries this is to have patience. Don't let the waiting period bring negative thoughts. Try this method and fulfil your dreams faster.

Chapter 4: History And Tradition Of Reiki

The roots of mindfulness can be traced back to the ancient times; to specifically about 5,000 years ago, although no written record on meditation has been enough to support this presumption. All the same, researchers suppose that our ancestors may have gained varied levels of heightened consciousness and experienced mindfulness while quietly gazing at their fire as it flickers.

The earliest written record on mindfulness includes those that originate from the tradition of Hinduism called Vedantism, dating back to 1500 BCE. By the 6th and 5th centuries BCE, the Taoists (China) and Buddhists (India) developed their own versions of meditation. In 500 BC, the teachings of Buddha, a highly prominent advocate of meditation, spread all over Asia and many other countries. Different cultures then adopted the mindfulness practice using their own methods.

In ancient religion, people practice meditation in the form of rhythmic, repetitive chant, known today as mantra. Mantras help you connect to the "spirit," which is the foundation of everything in this universe. These are a powerful tool that helps you focus your mind and eliminate all the distractions which might be in your surroundings. Over the centuries, meditation has evolved into a more structured practice which we enjoy and benefit from today.

How it Relates to Vipassana

Mindfulness is a variation of Vipassana, a traditional meditation practice derived from the Buddhist culture. Vipassana means insight or clear-seeing in Prakrit language and its origins date back to 6th century B.C. This practice stems from the Theravada Buddhism tradition which was popularized by S.N. Goenka, and the Vipassana Movement. Vipassana is also referred to as "mindfulness of breathing" and is known in the Western countries simply as "mindfulness." As it evolved, however, slight modifications to the practice have been created.

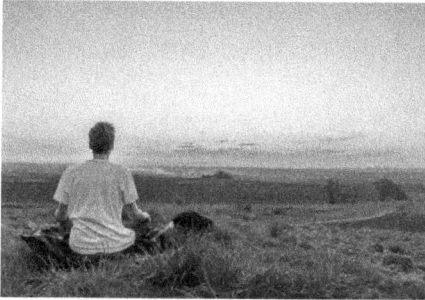

From East to West

Centuries after first becoming popular in the East, mindfulness reached the Western region of the globe and gained a number of followers by the middle of the 20th century. Experts started evaluating the effects of mindfulness and discovered its benefits during the 60s and 70s. In recent years, two mindfulness-based programs have been developed to help individuals suffering from stress and chronic depression, namely, Mindfulness-Based Stress Reduction (MBSR) and

Mindfulness-Based Cognitive Therapy (MBCT).

Jon Kabat-Zinn, along with his colleagues, developed the MBSR at the University of Massachusetts Medical School in 1979. The aim was to help individuals w ho all had a wide range of both mental and physical health problems, particularly those who are looking to decrease their stress levels. MBSR programs are intensive mental trainings that enable each participant to access his or her own resources in order to respond more effectively to pain, stress, illness, and other challenges of daily life.

MBSR has since been taught and further developed in clinics and hospitals for staff, patients, and medical students. It is also performed in prisons, companies, government agencies, inner-city areas, law firms, schools and universities. MBSR through this research has proven itself to be an effective remedy for depression, anxiety, life stress, chronic pain, fatigue, even cancer and psoriasis, among many other health conditions. It also provides a strong framework for self-care support.

Inspired by the success of the MBSR program, MBCT was developed in the UK by Professors Mark Williams and Zindel Segal and Dr. John Teasdale. It aims to help people who are vulnerable to depression relapse. Rumination, or the act of repetitively re-running negative thoughts in our minds, is the thinking pattern that often makes people susceptible to a depressive relapse. MBCT presents mindfulness skills that provide people with an alternative approach to rumination and its prevention. It is also meant to help prevent the buildup of negative thinking patterns that may result in a depressive relapse.

Currently, MBCT is among the treatments recommended in the National Institute of Clinical Excellence (NICE) guidelines for people who have gone through 3 or more bouts of depression. Further, the Mental

Health Foundation has launched an awareness campaign to help spread more information about, and increase people's access to, various mindfulness-based courses.

Myths About Mindfulness

Considering its long history and the progress it has made since it was first put to use, it is understandable for certain myths to crop up about what mindfulness is. This is one of the reasons why, despite having proven its benefits, many people still tend to be a bit cautious when they hear the term 'meditation' or 'mindfulness'. So, before moving any further, let us take a look at these myths and debunk them.

Mindfulness is not a religion.

At present, mindfulness is practiced by millions of people around the world, regardless of race, faith, or religion. Contrary to what some might believe, mindfulness (and meditation in general) is not a religion - it is a method of training the mind. Though many people who meditate are religious, many agnostics and atheists are keen meditators as well.

You don't always have to sit on the floor with your legs crossed.

Mindfulness meditation can also be practiced whilst the person is seated on a chair, a park bench, or the like. You may also bring mindful awareness to your everyday activities such as eating, taking a shower, walking at the park, speaking with other people, or simply sitting on your office chair.

Mindfulness does not take a great deal of time.

While it requires persistence and patience, meditation will not eat up a lot of your time. In fact, many meditators soon discover that mindfulness frees them from the pressure of time, and thus they have more to spend on other activities.

Mindfulness is not as complicated as it seems.

Mindfulness may seem difficult, but after each session, you get to understand the workings of the human mind a little better than before, especially your own. Not only does this create a better sense of self, it also enables you to become more understanding of others. As you progress with experience, going into the mindful state becomes almost effortless.

Mindfulness does not deaden the mind or interfere with lifestyle and career goals.

Mindfulness is not about being forced to accept the unacceptable. Rather, it is about perceiving the world in an entirely new manner; providing you with greater clarity which lets you make wiser, more pronounced decisions and actions to change the things that need be changed, and accept those that cannot be changed. Mindfulness helps cultivate a deeper, more compassionate awareness which will help you determine your life goals and enable you to discover the most ideal path towards realizing your earnest values.

Chapter 5: Getting To Know The Reiki Master

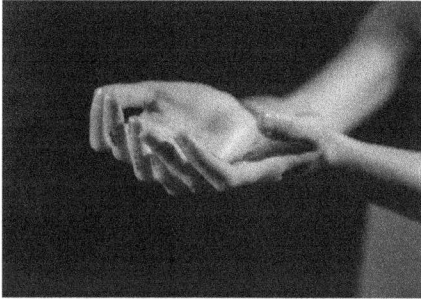

What Is A Reiki Master?

Given the idea of the ace level and the energies that become accessible to us, being a Reiki ace can be a progressing procedure including consistent self-improvement. With the ace attunement and the utilization of the ace image, we get the chance to open increasingly more totally to the boundless capability of this art and to create within each of us the characteristics that are held within the vitality of Reiki.

Consider every one of the parts of Reiki vitality - other than the possibility to mend for all intents and purposes all disease, it likewise contains boundless love, delight, harmony, empathy, astuteness, bounty and significantly more. We know these are the characteristics of Reiki on the grounds that individuals experience them when giving or accepting Reiki medications. They are particularly evident when we think about the wellspring of Reiki. When doing as such, many are lifted up into a protected spot where they feel totally thought about and become mindful of the superb potential outcomes that can emerge out of inside.

When we mull over these things it is anything but difficult to move toward becoming overpowered with good faith and the certain comprehension of the fact that any, and all, difficulties of the world can be overcome and that our existence could be a great encounter. The Japanese term of the highest degree in Reiki is

Shinpiden that signifies "Puzzle Teaching." The riddle that is talked about is the secret of God's adoration, shrewdness, and power.

It is a riddle since God has no limits; every one of the qualities of God including marvel, excellence, and elegance reach out a long way past our capacity to understand. Regardless of how created in this life or in any future degree of presence, we will never completely get it. This is the reason it is and will consistently stay a superb secret.

When we get the Usui ace image and the attunement that engages it, it makes the likelihood for us to end up mindful of the Ultimate Reality. This is communicated in the meaning of the Usui ace image that demonstrates that it speaks to that piece of the self that is as of now totally illuminated! When we utilize the ace image, we are really interfacing with our own edified selves. This truth be told, is the genuine wellspring of Reiki vitality - it really originates from the most profound and most significant piece of our own inclination, our very own illuminated self. Even though we might be under the impression that this phenomenon is originating from afar and descends to use through the crown chakra, the fact of the matter is that it is merely a hallucination and just shows up along these lines in light of our restricted mindfulness.

The healing energy that is summoned in Reiki is bestowed upon by the creator. It is therefore this energy that leads us to heal and opens us up to greater self-understanding and enlightenment. However, improvement doesn't happen naturally. Reiki regards our through and through freedom and doesn't compel advancement on us, yet on the off chance that we look for it and expect it, and use Reiki for this reason, at that point absolutely, we will be guided into a more prominent recuperating background. Attempt this analysis. Begin by conducting

Reiki on your own self utilizing our ace image in the hands within a position which is agreeable. (On the off chance that you aren't an ace at Reiki but rather at the first or second level, attempt it in any case without the ace image.) Then ruminate over this insistence. "I give up totally to the Reiki vitality and the source from which it comes." Repeat this assertion again and again, at that point as the Reiki vitality keeps on streaming, with your inward eye, search for the wellspring of Reiki, either inside yourself or above.

By doing this, you will have numerous significant encounters. These are probably going to incorporate ending up progressively mindful of the way Reiki functions inside you and sensing that its astonishing characteristics. New conceivable outcomes for self-awareness will be exhibited and you will be welcome to partake in life in a progressively important manner. As your mindfulness draws much nearer to the actual source, you will wind up mindful of stunning bits of knowledge and have regularly expanding encounters of happiness, security, and harmony. This is a superb exercise and definitely justified even despite the time. We recommend you do this regularly and as you do as such, these encounters will end up more grounded. At that point, on the off chance that you acknowledge the mending changes that are displayed, profound recuperating will start occurring and you will likewise start accepting direction about how to improve your life. While this contemplation is basic, it is additionally exceptionally ground-breaking and can lead you into a cheerful and sound perspective, making enduring changes that will shape the establishment of an increasingly advantageous life.

Reiki can manage you in approaches to make its recuperating power progressively advantageous and to mend all the more profoundly. What's more, simultaneously, one can assume that this discipline will direct you to additional mending strategies which are actually directly available for your use notwithstanding Reiki. You may likewise get direction about changes you have to make that expect you to make a move. Your capacity to settle on choices can improve, making it extremely simple to choose precisely what you need, who to connect with, where to work, and so on and this could bring about a totally new course for your life!

When you are engaged with the recuperating procedure, a great method to decide your advancement is to utilize your external world as a sign of your internal improvement. This works since we show our whole experience through our contemplations and goals - both cognizant and oblivious. When we experience something in our lives, it is on the grounds that some piece of our being has made it. When we acknowledge this thought and assume total liability for what happens in our lives, we enter an extremely amazing spot. We would then be able to get rid of the things which do not provide any benefit and make every part of our lives better.

In the event that your external world contains positive encounters, and you are making a mind-blowing most, this implies your internal world is in a comparative state. The turn around is likewise valid, thereby when we go through agonizing experiences and circumstances, or are disillusioned or experience by situations that cultivate dread, stress or uncertainty, this is additionally in light of the fact that some piece of our inward being is out of parity and necessities recuperating. On the off chance that something upsetting, or undesirable happens in your life, instead of accusing other individuals or conditions outside yourself, direct your consideration internally and search for the piece of yourself that has made this terrible occasion. At that point utilize your Reiki mending abilities to support and recuperate this part. When you do this, the disagreeable encounters will stop and be supplanted by sound positive encounters.

As we proceed on our recuperating way, we will end up mindful of a degree of cognizance that lives profoundly inside every one of us that can bring a great better approach for living. It makes another disposition that is totally positive and carries with it the capacity to take care of numerous issues and make positive outcomes that beforehand we didn't think conceivable.

What Are the Roles Of A Reiki Master?

There are numerous individuals looking for recuperating who wonder, what do Reiki Masters do, what is the job of a Reiki Master healer and what would they be able to assist me with?

These are on the whole extremely significant inquiries to pose. For customers of Reiki, yet in addition for Reiki Masters themselves. Numerous recently prepared

Reiki Master healers, and even many experienced experts and educators, don't have a reasonable comprehension about their job as a healer.

Understanding the job a Reiki Master plays in taking an interest in your mending is significant for everybody included. Understanding what a Reiki Master does and doesn't do impacts a mending session and otherworldly and self-awareness. For the customer, however for the Reiki Master healer as well.

So, what does a Reiki Master do precisely? It might shock you, yet a Reiki Master isn't required to fix your medical issues! From my own encounters working with customers all through the world, I have seen that numerous individuals don't completely comprehend the job a Reiki Master healer plays with regards to mending. There is a constant flow of customers who go to a Reiki Master with a rundown of desires.

Reiki Master healers just associate you with The Source. Regardless of whom your Reiki Master healer is, their job is to associate your body, being and vitality with the vitality of The Source. From here, it is up to The Source what gets mended in you and what doesn't. The aftereffects of a Reiki treatment are not the duty of the healer. Some portion of the duty rests with the customer and the rest with The Source. So how open the customer is to being mended, the amount they have confidence in the capacity to recuperate, and that they are so associated with God, The Source, are a portion of the numerous elements that decide the achievement of a mending session. It is the job of your Reiki Master to associate your vitality with the vitality of The Source. From that point, a customers mending is about their more profound association with The Source.

The principal obligation is to oneself, to sustain and create from inside, and to discharge any cynicism from inside.

Regularly in this day and age, we run over a clash that we can decide to either accept or smoothly resolve. We may get malady that we are to mend from comprehensively. We are tested with negative passionate responses that we should relinquish. We are tested with remaining negative feelings from quite a while ago, sentiments; for example, stress, outrage, low self-esteem, we are not to enable these emotions to rot and develop however to release them and recuperate. Most importantly, we need to deal with ourselves, living by the Reiki Principles as given by Mikao Usui, the originator of Reiki, and permitting ourselves Reiki mending each day. All things considered; we are not very useful to any other individual in the event that we are ourselves a wreck! I find that for myself and for other Reiki Masters, this first duty is the hardest to complete. It is a continuous exertion that gets simpler with long stretches of training. The key is to prop up back to the lessons of Usui with a receptive outlook and humble soul.

The subsequent obligation is to individuals who come to us for Reiki. There are individuals from the open who want treatment and understudies who seek commencement and educating.

When somebody seeks a treatment with Reiki, my instructing was to disclose to the customer that Reiki is a comprehensive vitality, going to where it is most required, and to urge the customer to comprehensively deal with their wellbeing. Reiki works uniquely in contrast to allopathic prescription. While allopathic drug fixes the side effect, Reiki mending is aimed at the entire individual. For example, if a customer came griping of knee torment, it might be that the knee is focused on in light of the fact that the hip is twisted. The hip may have turned into that path so as to make up for a shoulder being twisted. This may have occurred because of worry in the individual's life. On the off chance that this pressure is as yet progressing, the Reiki is probably going to mend the pressure first. This bodes well, as leaving the worry there may prompt further bear hip-knee misalignment and further knee harm! Some portion of the duty of the Reiki Master is to make the customer mindful of this all-encompassing procedure and the requirement for a few sessions. This allows the Reiki to recuperate the side effects just as the hidden causes.

At the point when an understudy seeks commencement and educating, this is the start of a profound, passionate, mental and physical adventure. The Reiki Master needs to consider the street went before this point and above all, bolster the understudy on their energizing new venture with Reiki.

A significant number of us have come into Reiki from a foundation of physical or passionate agony. For a few, there was a profound void to fill. A decent Reiki Master will be delicate to the necessities of their understudies. This implies staying away from natural aggravations in the class to think about understudies with compound sensitivities. It means relinquishing injurious comments given by furious spirits. It means being firm yet delicate with understudies from a sincerely despondent life. Most importantly, in the class, the Reiki Master ought to guarantee the understudy feels needed, regarded, acknowledged and adored. After the commencement and educating, the Reiki Master can bolster their understudy by making accessible and focusing on the requirement for ordinary contact and supervision. The rest is up to the understudy and what feels directly for their advancement with Reiki.

The third obligation is towards friends and family and every single other animal; to put it plainly, our condition. Our mending incorporates thinking about this condition.

This doesn't mean enabling an injurious relative to manhandle us or adding to social wrongs since every other person appears to! It means being capable, cherishing genuinely, and enabling recuperating to stream any place it is required and with the consent of the healer. For example, a Reiki Master can begin every day by asking that they are a channel, or course, for Reiki vitality and enabling it to stream any place they stroll in nature. A Reiki Master can buy earth amicable items. A Reiki Master can be accessible for relatives for recuperating as feels fitting and be a power for good. A Reiki Master living by the Reiki Principles will win their living truly, respect their educators and older folks, and be charitable to each living thing.

One of the most normally looked for after administrations I offer to customers is relationship mending. Regardless of who the individual and what kind of life they live, everybody has associations with individuals. Regardless of whether with an accomplice, a companion, a relative or a business associate, a huge piece of life comes down to the connections we have with others. So, relationship recuperating is a prevalent region that individuals frequently need assistance with. Anyway, numerous individuals expect a Reiki Master to do something amazing and power two individuals together in 'amicability'. This is a remarkable inverse of concordance. Indeed, utilizing vitality to constrain two individuals together is more much the same as dark enchantment than mending. No Reiki Master should utilize vitality diverting to control the Will of someone else. Regardless of what the goal might be. There are significant explanations behind why individuals meet up. There are similarly significant purposes behind why individuals part. Inside this uniting and separating of connections are numerous significant open doors for self-advancement and otherworldly development.

So, the job of a Reiki Master isn't to conflict with the regular progression of the Universe. The job of a Reiki Master is to help the individuals in a relationship to make harmony with their connections, to comprehend the message, if conceivable, and to enable them to mend and proceed onward if that is the regular course that relationship should take. The best job a Reiki Master could accept that is turning into a channel and manual for assistance individuals comprehend the more profound importance of their connections. The specialty of Reiki and profound recuperating plans to enable the individual to rehearse it. By figuring out how your condition communicates with you, and how you cooperate with your condition, you can start to utilize your musings, goal, feeling, and vitality as instruments of progress. Now and again, numerous customers have an ordinary Reiki Master healer who mends them, yet they don't wish to learn Reiki themselves. We have a couple of customers who feel this way. Anyway, there are various hindrances to this that customers ought to know about.

The job of a Reiki Master is to recuperate, enable and improve their customers. In the event that a co-dependent relationship creates among healed and healer, this can be counter-productive for the development and advancement of the customer. By not figuring out how you make vitality at each minute, how you channel it into your life, and how your life turns into an impression of that vitality you channel, you will never arrive at the purpose of being responsible for your heading throughout everyday life. Acknowledge how vitality streams and you can accomplish self-dominance. There is little reason in a Reiki Master healer expelling a negative vitality hinders from inside you if your considerations, expectations, and activities are more than once re-making those equivalent blockages. When you figure out how you make these vitality squares yourself, and you find how to discharge them yourself, there is no compelling reason to contract a Reiki Master to recuperate you. Since you can do it without anyone else's help. The best job a Reiki Master can take is spurring you to change. Since without change, there is no genuine advancement. The vitality of Reiki itself will help change to happen naturally. Anyway, by learning Reiki, you enable that change to turn out to be a lot further and unquestionably increasingly significant.

Chapter 6: The Power Of Reiki

Reiki is one of the most powerful medical alternatives used to effectively boost health and well-being. It has the ability to rebalance body systems to instantly relieve pain and also works as a preventive therapy. This healing process is non-invasive, and its effects are long term. Reiki healing can ease conditions like high blood pressure, headaches, and arthritis just to name a few. During a Reiki session performed by a professional, a patient can have an increased flow of life force from the power of unleashing energy. Reiki's composition represents many new possibilities to come. Reiki healing has been successful for many different health issues, from depression to weight loss, maintaining focus, increasing strength and empowering confidence while at the same time improving healthy bodies.

Call for Peace! (30 Minutes)

Find a comfortable space, dim the lights and light some candles. Lay down if you can, though sitting is fine, and close your eyes.

Clear your mind and think about just breathing in and breathing out, and relax each time as you do so.

Each time you exhale, count down from five to one. Relax more and more with each exhalation. Focus only on your breathing and counting down.

When you reach six complete exhales, you should be completely relaxed and only think about your breath.

Picture yourself walking slowly along a well-kept gravel path.

You can see your feet with each step and hear the soft shuffle of the gravel below.

Concentrate on each step you are taking and notice your feet as you walk.

You feel relaxed and optimistic.

As the path stretches out in front of you, you can see the hills far ahead.

It is fall, and the leaves are falling.

Imagine that you can smell the dried and yet still colorful leaves along the path.

Your mind is calm, and your vision is clear.

The rhythm of your walk is soothing. The sound of the gravel is soft. It is only interrupted by the songs of the birds.

They are calling messages to each other. What could they be saying?

Most are small songbirds, and you should imagine they are fluttering by. Picture what they look like, what they smell like and what they sound like. They are getting ready for a long flight, and you are wondering where they will be going.

The air is so fresh and clean, and you are walking, walking, walking. You try to make every step the same and make every sound a rhythm in your mind.

It is cool outside, but you are warm.

You are totally relaxed, and your pace is effortless.

Your arms are moving in silent motion and in sync with your steps.

The path seems an endless journey, turning and moving.

It almost feels as if you are still and the path is moving beneath you – carrying you, protecting you.

Your mind is clear and relaxed, and your body is renewed and filled with energy.

Chapter 7: Common Ailments To Heal With Reiki

As you have already seen in Chapter 7: Benefits and Limitations of Reiki, there are quite a few ways that Reiki can heal the common ailments. You may still be wondering how it's possible for a Reiki healing session to heal someone of these various ailments and degrees of unhealthiness. Here are some of the key points to remember how Reiki works and why it is possible:

Reiki asks permission to work on the areas of a person that need the most attention. When you are going to a Reiki practitioner regularly, Reiki will guide the healer to the right position for healing work. If the issue is chronic, then the problem will work itself out over time as Reiki is applied often and frequently to help rebalance the generally positive and light flow of energy into these areas.

Chronic conditions, including cancer, are not just physical; they are the build up over time of negative and low vibrational energy that can come from a variety of sources.

Reiki balances the chakras and as you have read, each chakra aligns with specific body systems, emotions, thoughts and other energies. When the energy of these areas is shifted and purged, or cleansed with healing Reiki energy, it sets in motion a general healing of all systems.

Reiki only works if you use it, so if you actually want to cause healing and reduce chronic problems, or eradicate them, you have to apply Reiki as often as possible in order to treat the ailment.

Reiki is a channeled energy that comes through the Reiki practioner into the client. The Reiki will guide the practitioner to where they need to go in order to resolve the issue.

Bodies are not just flesh and blood and bone; they are many layered and one of the greatest misunderstandings in the medical community is that you can't expect to heal someone's whole body system with prescription drugs and surgery.

Men, women, and people of every age are able to benefit form Reiki as a healing resource and when it is carefully applied to a certain disorder or ailment, it will result in a broad and general healing, as well as a specific and pin-pointed healing that cannot be seen through x-rays, or MRI scans, but can be felt emotionally, mentally, spiritually, and often physically.

All of these practical examples of what Reiki is capable of demonstrates that there are numerous factors at play in any healing process and that in order to try and operate your energy at optimal capacity, you have to evolve your energy to be at a higher vibrational frequency.

You can change your frequency in other ways, including diet, exercise, hobbies and passions, music, dancing, creativity, sex, love, and so forth. There are a lot of things that can change our vibration and energy and they can either be low or high frequency.

Reiki is pure light and high vibrational and so if you are wanting to change the energy of your low energy and remove blocks and obstacles to flowing freer and higher, then Reiki is a quick and easy way to explore and experience those results.

There are a number of methods for healing all of these ailments and you have already read about what they are in this book. You can begin to practice them when you are attuned to the degrees of Reiki you desire to learn and can begin your healing journey NOW!

Here are more of the possibilities for healing with Reiki:

Physical Conditions and Wellness

Allergies and recurring colds

Anemia

Autoimmune conditions (Sjogren's syndrome, celiac disease)

Circulation and cardiovascular health (arteriosclerosis, angina)

Diabetes and regulation of blood sugar levels

Inflammatory issues and disorders (gout, rheumatoid arthritis, etc.)

Menopause

Fertility and childbirth issues or health

Thyroid issues

Hormonal imbalances

Liver disease

Various forms of cancer and post-cancer treatment recovery

AIDS and HIV

Recovery form surgery

Prevention of surgery

Lymphatic flow

Mental / Emotional Conditions and Wellness

Anxiety and stress disorders

Bipolar syndrome

Phobias

Post-traumatic stress disorder

Panic attacks

Smoking cessation

Drug and alcohol addictions/ substance abuse

Heartache and heartbreak

Grief and loss

Fear

Worry

Insomnia and sleep disorders

Repressed emotions

Inner child healing

Self-esteem and self-worth

Self-control

Cognitive abilities

Memory recall

Autism

Neurodegenerative disorders (Parkinson's, Alzheimer's, dementia)

Spiritual Conditions and Wellness

Spiritual abundance

Prosperity

Inner richness

Life purpose and personal truth

Life goals and ambitions determined and realized

Existential crisis

Past life and karmic healing

Kundalini Awakening

Astral travel, or astral projection

Psychic abilities opened and enhanced

Clairvoyance/ claircognizance

Visions, nightmares and lucid dreaming

Processing the opening of the chakras, leading to spiritual awakening

Collective Consciousness

The lists are endless because with Reiki, you can heal just about anything. If you are working to become a Reiki practitioner or Master, it is important to ask your client through the initial intake process before a session, what current medical conditions, if any, they may currently have. Being well-informed about what your client is going through is important, and even though Reiki is a safe tool for healing that will not cause an issue with an existing condition, you may want to work alongside whatever current medical needs they are having and open to sharing with you before their session.

All of these ailments and conditions are accounts of real experiences that people have reported healing and even curing after a consistent program of regularly scheduled Reiki healing treatments. There is no way to cure anything with just one session, and so if you are looking for a cure, then you must be prepared to do the work. And as for the practitioner, if you are helping someone on their healing journey, patience is a virtue.

Chapter 8: Reiki Attunement Ceremony

Reiki is such an amazing form of energy work and can benefit people on so many levels that becoming a Reiki practitioner seems like an easy decision. It can be, for many people!

However, sometimes understanding more of what is involved in becoming a Reiki practitioner can help with the decision. Becoming a Reiki practitioner does involve study, practice, and some minor lifestyle changes.

Even though every human has a connection to universal energy and Reiki energy, that energy may not be accessible or there may be interference with the connection. Through your studies as a Reiki practitioner, you will become a pure conduit for the Reiki energy. Just like keeping your body clear from mind-altering substances, your body needs to be opened and cleared in order to properly channel Reiki energies.

Once Attuned to the different levels of Reiki, those Attunements last a lifetime. You do not need to get re-attuned regularly, or ever, once you receive the different levels. However, practicing Reiki regularly will ensure that you continue to be a clear conduit for the Reiki energy. Attunements don't fade or grow weaker, but it is like any muscle or skill, the more it is used and practiced, the more fluent the energy becomes.

Attunement Ceremony

Anyone can learn Reiki. Anyone can become a Reiki practitioner. Why not, it is such a powerful tool for healing and amazing service to offer. The journey to becoming a Reiki practitioner does involve study and practice. Along the path to become a Reiki practitioner, there is a ceremony that every new initiate must go through every time they advance a level in their training.

This ceremony is called an Attunement. The Reiki Attunement ceremonies are performed on a practitioner after they go through the course material for Reiki Level I, then after they go through the material and study for Reiki Level II, and again once a practitioner reaches the Master Level.

For Reiki Level I there are four Attunements that must be received from a Reiki practitioner. It is recommended that all your attunements come from the same teacher, or at least your Attunements for each level come from the same teacher.

Every person is already connected to Reiki and the energies of the universe. Going through the Attunement ceremonies helps the practitioner's body-mind clear so it can become a pure channel for Reiki and healing.

With the Attunement ceremonies, some teachers will perform all the Level I Attunements in one ceremony while others may do separate ceremonies for each one.

Before receiving your Level I attunements, you'll want to prepare yourself. Some preparations are only recommended, however they can definitely enhance the attunement process and make for a better and more profound experience.

Keeping the body free of alcohol and mind-altering substances for up to twenty-four hours before an Attunement is recommended for the same reasons as it is recommended for keeping the body clear prior to performing a session. Energy flows better and freer through a clean and clear conduit. Any substance that alters the mind can inhibit that flow.

Prescription medication that has been prescribed by a health care professional should not be interrupted for an Attunement ceremony.

Another way to keep the body clean and clear is to be conscious of what you are eating and drinking, especially twenty-four hours prior to the Attunement ceremony.

What that means is eating and drinking clean, whole foods, such as whole grains, fruits, vegetables, legumes, nuts, seeds, eggs, and clean meats. Avoiding processed foods, processed sugars, and artificially flavored, processed and sweetened drinks, especially soda.

Stored energy and energy blocks that build up from mild altering recreational substances and unclean, processed foods can inhibit the energetic flow during an Attunement. Even just removing those substances from your diet and routine for the day before an Attunement can enhance the experience.

Another recommended preparation is to meditate every day for a week leading up to your Attunement ceremony. Meditation will help clear your body and mind as a conduit to receive your Attunements. Even just meditating the day before and the day of your Attunements can help your body-mind shift into that vibration for the Attunements.

Reiki Attunements are an important part of the Reiki journey. They can be performed in person or at a distance. If your Reiki teacher lives far away and is teaching at a distance, then receiving the Attunements from a distance is equally as powerful as getting them in person.

After your Attunements, keep working through your course material as called. Progress onto the next Reiki Level II course material as you feel comfortable.

Depending on the course you are taking, you may be required to complete certain tasks before moving onto the next level. Many courses include a regiment of 21 consecutive days of self-Reiki treatments, to simulate the twenty-one days Usui spent meditating on the mountain. Other courses stick primarily to written material and yet others might even have an exam of some kind to complete. Make sure to thoroughly complete the tasks and course work before moving on.

During the Ceremony

Every single person experiences Reiki Attunements and Reiki energy differently. If you've never received an Attunement before, or if you have, having a journal or piece of paper handy to document your experiences is recommended.

Your Reiki teacher will perform a ceremony that includes the Reiki symbols that Dr. Usui rediscovered during his meditation and study. Each ceremony is set for the highest good of the student receiving the Attunement. The energy is intended to strengthen the student's connection to Reiki and universal energy.

Think of the body as a radio. There are different radio stations that operate on different frequencies to broadcast different kinds of information. In terms of the body, a Reiki Attunement changes the frequency in which the body operates so that it can better receive and broadcast Reiki energy.

The Attunement will allow you to access and use Reiki energy whenever you would like, sort of like programming a phone number on speed dial. You become a clear, strong receiver for the Reiki energy after an Attunement whereas before you are only able to pick up trace information.

A full Attunement process can last about twenty to thirty minutes, usually.

For an in-person Attunement, your Reiki teacher will likely have you sit in a chair and they will perform the ceremony on you.

When receiving and attunement in person, the Attunement is performed in silence. The student should also keep their eyes closed for the ceremony.

If you are receiving a distance Attunement, your Reiki teacher should establish a set time and date that the Attunement will be performed. When your time comes, make sure you are relaxed and sitting, or lying down, in a comfortable space. You can light candles, burn incense, or find other ways to enhance the ambiance of your space.

Playing music or entering a meditative state can also be helpful during a Reiki Attunement.

During an Attunement, it is best to turn off all phones or personal electronics, or at least set them in a different room or across your room. Electronic frequencies can interfere with Reiki energy and Attunements. Plus, decreasing distractions is ideal when receiving such Attunements.

Many students have received both in-person and distance Attunements, based on who they are learning each Level from, or if they retake a course for review, and report that the experiences between an in-person Attunement and a distance Attunement aren't that different. Some have even said that distance Attunements feel more powerful than an in-person ceremony.

It is not uncommon to experience visions or images and sensations during an Attunement ceremony. Some students will completely fall asleep. This is not a bad thing. Falling asleep doesn't mean the Attunement didn't work.

Sometimes students don't feel anything at all during an Attunement. Again, this doesn't mean that the ceremony didn't work. Not experiencing sensations or visions doesn't mean that the shifts in your energetic vibration and frequencies didn't take. Some students just experience a far more subtle shift. There is no right or wrong way to experience a Reiki Attunement.

Some common sensations include feelings of cold, heat, tingling, or a pulling sensation in various parts of the body. Other times there can be an emotional response, such as crying or other strong emotional feelings. Students have been known to see images, sometimes clear and meaningful, other times scattered and less precise.

Level I Reiki consists of 4 different Attunements. Level II Reiki includes and Attunement to the Reiki symbols. Then the

Master Level includes an Attunement to the Master Reiki Symbol.

Some teachers have you go through the entire course and then do all the Attunements at once. Other teachers perform all the Attunements once you get to the end of Level I Reiki, but still require you to go through the course work. There are many different ways to receive your Attunements and there is no one formula for how a teacher might perform them.

With each Attunement, energy is released from the student's body that is creating blocks or altering the energetic frequency. The energy that is released during an Attunement shifts your body back to a more natural, receptive frequency.

After a Level I Attunement you can work on yourself with Reiki energy. When you complete the Level II course and receive that Attunement and learn your symbols, you can work on yourself and others with Reiki energy. After receiving your Master Level Attunement you learn a Master

Symbol and learn how to Attune other students to Reiki.

It is a personal choice on how far you want to progress in Reiki. Not all Reiki students become Reiki Masters. Some students stop at Level I Reiki and others stop at Level II Reiki. You may decide to progress to a certain point and then stop. Then you could receive a calling to move to the next level several years later, or not.

The level of Reiki that you progress to may simply be based on what your goal is with using Reiki. Do you want to start a Reiki Practice and provide paid services to clients? Do you want to incorporate it into another form of healing such as massage or nursing? Do you want to become a Reiki teacher and pass on Reiki to other students?

Think about those questions before you decide how far you want to take your Reiki study.

Reiki Attunements work similarly to a Reiki session. While you are receiving an

Attunement, your body is taking in the Reiki energy that it needs. The body intuitively knows and draws in how much energy it needs and what shifts need to be made within the body for success.

Your body-mind isn't participating in the Attunement process. The Bodymind uses the Reiki energy during your Attunement to observe what aspects within your body are not serving you to the highest good. Once those aspects are identified your body can release and shift those energies to where they need to be.

Self-treatments after an Attunement are important to keep these shifts and releases in place, giving your body time to adjust and then remain in that shifted state.

Originally, the concept behind separating the Attunements out and performing separate ceremonies was in an attempt to ensure that a Reiki student wanted to go through the complete course and the different Reiki Levels. However, receiving the additional Attunements at the same time does not mean a student is required to finish their course study if they change their mind.

Additionally, if a student decides to take a brush-up course later, or wants to get back into Reiki, most teachers require students who are rediscovering Reiki or have taken a sabbatical to start from the beginning and receive their Attunements again.

The belief that a student can only handle one Attunement at a time is limiting to the mind and body's Reiki journey. Fortunately, times are progressing and it is becoming more accepted that the body can, in fact, handle all Attunements at once if that is how the teacher wishes to give them.

After the Ceremony

Once the Attunement ceremony is complete, you might notice changes in your body immediately. Sometimes students get up from an Attunement and immediately start to feel the energy in their hands. This can be in the form of heat or a tingling sensation.

The energy can come on immediately, or for some students, they won't feel it until later. Sometimes a recently Attuned student won't feel that energy current until they go to perform their first Reiki session on themselves or someone else.

The energy that is constantly around us is unmeasurable by human standards. Our bodies aren't equipped to see thermal energy or hear certain waves of sound energy. We can only perceive certain types and amounts of energy at any given time. While you practice Reiki, you may begin to feel energy more strongly over time or experience it different ways, such as in visions or other manifestations of energy.

The more you practice, the more your body can perceive Reiki energy.

Other effects of getting Attuned to Reiki might include your hands heating up or tingling if you are around someone who could use a Reiki treatment. Your entire body might feel the heat, or cold when you are around someone who needs a session. There are many ways your body can feel and experience Reiki energy. It can take some time to understand what you are feeling and refine the meanings of what you are feeling.

If you are new to energy work and Reiki, this process can take longer. Some students who have previous experience with other kinds of energy work or bodywork, such as massage, or have spent time meditating and studying energy might have an easier time understanding and refining what they are feeling.

Everyone learns and adapts at their own pace. Take your time to really understand what it is that your body feels. Write it down and see if that helps you decipher the meanings.

If any of the sensations you feel or experience are uncomfortable, try taking a deep, calming breath and set an intention for yourself that you allow Reiki energy to flow freely through you. That discomfort can be caused by the energy flowing but not releasing properly.

After your Attunements, your body-mind continues to release energies that do not serve your highest good. Attunements powerfully heal your mind, body, and spirit. They also activate the seven chakras (more on chakras and energetic anatomy in later chapters).

Some students do not experience any noticeable shifts right away after receiving their Attunements. One idea is to surrender your body and mind to the changes, opening yourself up to the effects of the Attunement. This can help release any blockages that are slowing the Attunement shifts down.

You might even experience some symptoms of a physical body cleanse or detoxification process. Again, this is normal as your body's energy is shifting and sometimes physically shedding what no longer serves it.

During this time, it is important to listen to your body. It is always important to listen to your body, but especially after receiving an Attunement that is designed to shift your energetic frequencies.

If your body wants you to rest and take it easy, do that. If your body wants you to hydrate, make sure you do so. If you feel like you want to be outside in nature, adhere to that calling.

After every attunement, it is important to perform self-treatments on yourself daily. This is a good habit to get into even when you aren't going through a Reiki course or receiving Attunements.

Self-Treatments will be discussed in further detail in a later chapter, however, here is a brief overview. A self-Reiki treatment doesn't have to be long or include hand positions. They can, however, if you are doing daily self-treatments (as you should be), setting 30 to 45 minutes aside can seem unrealistic for some people.

So, performing a quick ten to fifteen-minute self-treatment is an easy workaround. These shorter treatments can be done while you are sitting at your desk, while eating dinner, or when you are lying down getting ready for bed. They don't necessarily require a ceremony or set up.

Holding your hands in an open position for ten minutes is an acceptable self-treatment. If you meditate daily, incorporate a self-treatment session into your mediation. You might find that it greatly enhances the meditation experience as well.

Drinking plenty of water will also encourage better energy flow. Some students experience headaches after Attunements or treatments. Drinking water can help reduce the probability of a headache.

After Attunements it is not uncommon to have vivid dreams or experience memories and emotions that you may have repressed, or not had cause to think of for some time. Trust your body-mind and encourage yourself to process these memories and emotions to heal. Continued mediation and self-treatments will also increase your ability to heal and process this information.

Once you have received your Attunements, continue to develop your Reiki skills. What separates Reiki from other energy work is that Reiki isn't sent. It is drawn into the client or recipient through the practitioner or conduit. If you continue to remind yourself of this while progressing through your studies, you will become a more skilled healer.

Since the practitioner is being in the session and not performing the session, no personal energy is used from the practitioner as they perform a treatment. After a session, practitioners can feel energized and maybe even feel some of the effects of the Reiki energy as it was drawn through them. Because the Reiki energy flow is one way, practitioners can't accidentally 'take on' or 'absorb' their client's pain, illness, or energy blockages.

The more you develop your Reiki skills, the more your intuition should develop as well. Just because you complete the course and receive your Attunements doesn't mean you should stop studying or improving your Reiki practice. There is always more to learn and you can always become a more proficient Reiki Healer.

Chapter 9: Awakening Your Higher Self

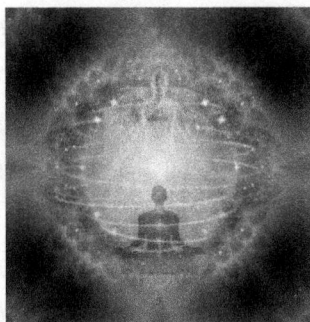

There is one topic we must discuss in order for everything else to make sense, and that is the idea of a higher self. We touched for a moment on this in Chapter 1, with the idea of our third eye, or our sixth sense. Let's explore this a little bit further.

The higher self is innate in every living thing. It has been called many things, including gut feelings and intuition, our soul, our spirit. To the untrained person, the higher self is an intangible thing. We cannot necessarily see it, hear it or physically feel it, but it is still there. When you have an inkling that something isn't quite right, or if you make a decision based on a gut feeling that may have no other logic, this is your higher self, guiding you in the right direction.

The good news is, we can be trained to become more in touch with our higher self. In fact, when we really look at it, our higher self is tangible after all. We can feel it, sense it, but only if we try. Imagine that this higher self is simply a small ball of energy that lives within us. For many spiritual followers, we know that our spiritual being will eventually leave our bodies in death, and leave to other parts of the universe. No matter what religion you follow, if any at all, this idea transcends all. Religion is based on this idea, and we see it playing out in varying degrees of heaven, and places in which our spirit will be free from the flesh. We cannot simply imagine that our consciousness will not go on once our bodies have expired.

This ball of energy, our higher self, has a mind all its own. It is our guiding energy that knows right from wrong and knows our true path. Think for a moment about the state of your life. Think about your career, your family, how you choose to live your life. Are you content with everything, or are there other things that you strive for? Do you feel you are in line with your conscience, or is there a nagging feeling in the back of your mind that is pulling you in a different direction?

This feeling is with everyone, and there is nothing wrong with following it, as it is simply your higher self, trying to tell you something. Our society has fallen far from a once virtuous place in which everyone followed their inner voices and did what was best for them, for their communities and the earth they call home. Instead, the world is filled with greed, money, and the pursuit of a 'stable' life filled with inanimate objects like fancy homes and cars that bring 'happiness.' In reality, we do not need any of those things to survive, and listening to your true self will help you distinguish what is necessary and what is greedy.

Many of us try and push these feelings away, as society is telling us what we need. Our desire to follow the crowd and do what is socially acceptable has imprisoned our spirits into endless days of work and responsibility that is slowly killing our energy. We often push our desires down to go to a tireless yet well-paying job to make money and live a responsible life, all the while reducing our higher self to nothing.

Instead, if we learn to work with our higher self, we unlock the potential of endless bounds of energy, happiness, and life. Our higher self, that little ball of energy within us, holds the key to a fulfilling life, one that may not be so prosperous monetarily, but one that is worth living in the end. If we learn to follow our intuitions given by the higher self, everything we truly need will come to us when we need it.

Now for some training to get in line with our true self. Simply, we must learn to follow our gut instinct. Those little feelings of dread and cues for you to do certain things are your roadmap. Understand that stress, anxiety, and depression are symptoms of an unhappy inner self. Your energy is off balance, and something in your life is causing it. Instead of suppressing these feelings by medicating with sedatives and mood stabilizers or self-medicating with alcohol or other substances, embrace and explore these feelings. Something in your life isn't quite right, and finding out what it is and making changes is the key to balancing your energy and emotion. If you don't feel right, something is wrong. It is as simple as that.

We certainly would not recommend getting up and leaving your job and abandoning your current life, unless of course, this is the only way to find spiritual peace. Instead, take some time to really discover what your true path is by paying attention to those gut feelings and determining where it is they are telling you to go. You cannot expect to be good at being in-tune with your higher self immediately, so don't make any rash decisions until you become comfortable with its signals.

For example, if you have begun to dread going to work every day, it may not be because of the work, but because of the specific environment. You may enjoy that same work somewhere else and does not require a complete upheaval of your life. Maybe you just need to find work with another company to bring your balance back. Or, maybe you discover after switching jobs that your work is no longer fulfilling and finding something new is really what you need. Now may be the time to start looking into a new career, your true calling.

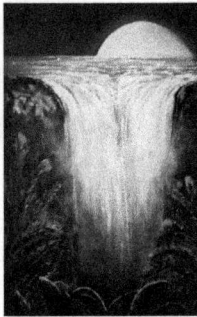

Remember that the universe will give you exactly what you need if you stop working on its energy. Everyone has a true path that they need to follow, one that brings ultimate happiness and joy. Once you are in line with this ideal energy path, everything will fall into place on its own. Going against this energy is like trying to swim up river after a heavy rain. You will fight the current but get nowhere. Giving in and flowing with the river will get you where you need to be faster. You simply need to accept that this river of energy knows where it is you need to be.

If you are someone that needs something to 'do,' trying keeping a journal expressing your feelings and emotions in relation to your situation. You can quickly develop feeling patterns in relation to specific events, like work, with certain people that take advantage of you, or even your location. Maybe you do better living in the country in the peace and quiet that on city streets. All of these things are valuable pieces of information that will be necessary for plotting out potential life changes.

If this doesn't sound like you, know that your inner self will give you the wisdom and energy you need to navigate this life, and it will guide you as it sees fit. This doesn't require careful planning, just the ability to tap into your true feelings and emotions at any given time. This doesn't mean that you won't make mistakes. You need to experience certain things to gain knowledge and wisdom to make the next step. You are not necessarily on the wrong path, and as long as you feel in-line with your true self, there is nothing to worry about.

Chapter 10: What Can Reiki Treat?

This is a controversial question within the reiki community, especially since there is no credible scientific data which supports any of their healing claims. Reiki was originally taught as a method of self-healing and self-care. The mastery of this ability gave those who healed themselves the power to heal others, and this is still the way it's viewed and taught.

Reiki does not officially claim to provide effective cures for any health problems. What it does is help people reconnect with universal life energy to ensure its proper flow throughout the body. When this energy flows naturally and in great strength, people enjoy health, vitality, and mental clarity. When its flow is blocked or weakened, the mind feels dull and the body becomes weak, making it vulnerable to sickness.

Practitioners receive the ability to manipulate this universal energy through a process known as attunement. This is received through proper training during a reiki learning course. Officially, one does not learn reiki, so much as receive it or relearn it.

If that sounds strange to you, you should understand that practitioners consider reiki to be a natural power. It's believed that this universal life energy is not an indifferent power, but an intelligent one that considers health and well-being to be the natural state.

According to this world view, illness is an unnatural state. What reiki practitioners do is encourage the body to return to its default condition—which is wholeness, balance, and vitality.

They can do so because this intelligent power guides them, an ability that is transferred through a practitioner to a novice. This power "attunes" the practitioner to their higher selves, allowing them to guide the energy through their hands. Those who learn reiki or receive its healing benefits become likewise attuned to their higher selves, and can therefore heal themselves and others.

Practitioners do not claim to cure disease, pain, fatigue, stress, or injury. Their function is to simply guide universal energy to those parts of the body where universal life energy is not flowing at optimum levels. Once they do that, the mind and body's natural healing abilities take over. In other words, reiki healing is a two-way process. Practitioners don't just manipulate energy which is believed to heal their patients. Patients must also take an active part in their own healing.

Supporters claim that reiki has healed anxiety, attention deficit disorders, cancer, chronic pain, Crohn's disease, depression, emotional distress, fatigue, various heart diseases, infertility, irritable bowel syndrome, neurodegenerative disorders, post-traumatic stress, and various other health issues. Please note that reiki does not claim to be a cure for these diseases.

Rather, it claims to have helped the body rid itself of them.

Chapter 11: Self-Esteem

Did you know that value, respect, and regard for self can easily describe self-esteem? These words make it easier to understand the term self-esteem and to understand it positively. Self-esteem is like medicine; an under-dose is as harmful as an overdose; it is at its best when it is somewhere in the middle. Too little of it can cause depression or feelings of defeat, while too much of it puts off other people and can cause harm to a personal relationship. People also make bad choices because of low self-esteem. What exactly is this self-esteem? Where do we get it from, and how can we train ourselves to strike a balance in the middle?

What Is Self-Esteem?

Self-esteem is a word that explains one's value or worth. It can be seen as how much you like and appreciate yourself. Self-esteem is enduring and stable; it reflects on a person's personality. It constitutes of personal beliefs and emotional states. Personal beliefs are like, "I am stupid" or "I am blessed," while emotional states are states like happiness, pride, triumph. Self-esteem is psychological, and it can predict some results like successful relationships, happiness, or even criminal behavior. Well, with that little information on self-esteem, we can see it is very crucial in our lives and plays a major role in success. Then where does self-esteem come from?

Our capabilities and value for self-form our self-esteem; this means that self-esteem comes from within us and from our thoughts. Self-esteem does not come from external forces, either family, friends, or your achievements. It means that no amount of support from family and friends can build your self-esteem, but tiny negative and positive thoughts of yourself can make and break your self-esteem respectively. We should also note that it is not only the thoughts on ourselves that affect our esteem but also the tiny thoughts on our capabilities that can build or break our self-esteem. It means that to improve our self-esteem, we should change how we think of ourselves and how we think of our capabilities. We should change our thoughts to be positive and start thinking highly of ourselves and our capabilities.

People with low self-esteem and their counterparts with positive self-esteem can be identified from a mile away as they show different distinct signs. A person's life experiences develop self-esteem. People with low self-esteem have gone through difficult life experiences like being ignored, teased, ridiculed, criticized harshly, or were sexually or emotionally abused. What are the signs of a person with low self-esteem?

· They view life negatively.
· They don't trust others.
· They have a perfectionist attitude.
· They are afraid of taking risks.

· They are afraid of being ridiculed.

· They depend on others to make decisions.

On the other hand, people with positive self-esteem show the following outward signs.

· They are confident.

· They are aware of their inner strengths.

· They are optimistic.

· They are problem-solvers.

· They are comfortable with different emotions.

· They trust others.

I know by now you are asking yourself, "Why is it so important to build on my self-esteem and maintain it? Well, ask no more; I got your back.

Importance of Self-Esteem

Now that we have an idea of what is self-esteem and how to achieve positive self-esteem let us find out what is the importance of it in our lives. Inner stability- Our bodies function like computers, and if we feed them 'bad input,' they give us back 'bad output.' When you value yourself more, your self-opinion goes up, and you stop being a people-pleaser.

When you love yourself, nature rewards you with a simple and light life.

Positive and steady self-esteem brings happiness.

Higher self-esteem gives you the ability to manage stress.

What is Not Self-Esteem?

We are living in an era where people equate recognition and wealth as self-esteem. Today's generation has no idea what self-esteem is, and if asked, they equate it to material things and achievements. We have already discussed what self-esteem entails, and right now, I want us to look at what it isn't.

· Self-esteem is not your net worth- We all know a person or two who equates their worth to their net worth. Some of us are not wealthy but live beyond our means to create an illusion that we are wealthy. Our material possessions are not a sign of your value as a human being.

· Self-esteem is not who you know- Some people depend on other people's opinion to know their value. Some even think that by dropping names of renowned people will earn admiration from others. We should understand that other people's opinions of us keep changing and no praises are enough to make us value ourselves.

· Self-esteem is not your appearance- Some people equate their self-esteem to their looks and the attention they attract. It is so unfortunate that this is what the media sells to us. Good looks are important, and they have their purpose in our lives, but they don't last forever. Your value should never be equated to something that has a life span. What happens when you start getting wrinkles or hair loss?

· Self-esteem is not what you do- Careers are good, and as much as they make us feel valuable, they should never determine our worth. To some people, their career is who they are. An end to that career will leave you feeling bad about yourself.

Obstacles of Self-Esteem

Self-esteem is the anticipation of positive results. As we said before, self-esteem is the value you place on self and not a personality trait. When you have positive self-esteem, you are motivated to work hard to devote resources and time towards achieving your goals. It is not self-esteem that brings you success; it is your efforts. Without self-esteem, you lack the self-drive to work towards achieving your goals. Here is a brief inventory of the obstacles of self-esteem.

· Critical authority figure

Is it possible to grow into a mature adult with positive self-esteem if you grew up being told that you are not good enough, and whatever you did wasn't either? No, children who grew up in critical homes; whose parents did not see anything positive in their actions have problems with self-esteem. It is difficult to value yourself if all you heard when you were growing up were words that told you otherwise. The shame enforced on you is blindingly painful.

· Uninvolved caregivers

It is not an easy task to motivate and convince yourself that you deserve better if your caregivers did not do that. Some parents have don't pay attention to their children's achievements, and when they do, they have no regard for them. Children who grow in such environments feel, forgotten, and unimportant. Such environments can make them feel unaccountable to any person, but that is postponed feelings from childhood. Unrecognized feelings can make a person believe that he/she has no value.

· Conflicts within the authority figures

In situations where parents or caregivers argue or fight a lot in front of their children, their children take in the distrustful conditions as a life model to them. Such threatening conflicts make the children feel responsible. Children carry those feelings of being contaminated into their adulthood. With such feelings, it is not easy to love and value yourself.

·Trauma

Sexual or emotional abuse is a big obstacle to self-esteem. People who have been subjected to such abusive experiences find it hard to trust themselves and hate the world. They blame themselves for the abuse and in an attempt to cope; they view themselves as shameful and repulsive. Such awful experiences hinder the growth of positive self-esteem.

Intellectualizing

In intellectualizing, you never involve your feelings or emotions in your thought, but you think of yourself in an intellectual and detailed way. You think and gauge yourself with regard to people's opinions or your success. For self-esteem to thrive well, you must involve your emotions; you must love yourself enough and think of yourself as a success and not a failure. Strong positive emotions should spark tiny thoughts about yourself.

· Negative self-talk

Some of us are too harsh on ourselves; we criticize ourselves a lot. Some people don't value themselves as much as they value others. Their concern for others is more than their own concern. You should be your cheerleader and avoid negative self-talk.

Roadblocks of Self-Esteem

Self-esteem is comprised of both your feelings and perception of yourself. Self-esteem is a journey of self-love and value of self. The journey to building your self-esteem begins with a spark of belief in yourself, and with time, you have the ability to love and value yourself. It is not an easy journey and just like any other journey out there. You will meet roadblocks along the way. Here are some roadblocks of self-esteem.

Comparison

In this digital age, it is common to feel like you are the only one failing in life. Applications like Facebook and Instagram gives us a peek at other people's life. Seeing some of our relatives and friends, good days can leave you feeling as if you are a failure. In social media, we only get to see only the best side of their life and little of the challenging parts. Also, the media packages its personalities as beautiful and fit, and they keep exaggerating. It gives 'normal' people a feeling that they are below standard and can't compete with what is out there. The media is always subjecting us to unfair comparisons every day.

Current relationships

Some relationships make us question ourselves. Sometimes, people make mean remarks about you and then act as if they were joking. You might also encounter discouragements from friends and family on your work or projects. Some will constantly tell you that you are not good enough, and they will never support you. Support from friends and family is important, and if you don't find it in them, you should limit your interactions with them. Surround yourself with people who will not block the growth of your self-esteem always. Self-esteem journey is not an easy one, especially to people with low self-esteem issues. You should not give up on this journey because of a few roadblocks here and there, but instead, you should fight throughout until you emerge a winner. The fruits of positive self-esteem are great; keep pushing.

Preparing for Your Walk

It is never too late to boost your self-esteem. As much as it is not an easy journey, it is doable and achievable. What can you do to raise your self-esteem? Here are some tips.

· Step outside- A little sunshine is good for every one of us. A little sunshine and especially when doing something active, can brighten our day. You can take a walk, simple gardening, or you can ride a bike.

· Accept your accomplishments- We should stop undermining our achievements and accept them. A pat on the back for a job well done can go a long way in boosting our esteem. We should stop criticizing ourselves and focus on positive thinking.

· Power pose- I could not also believe that a mere power pose can boost our self-esteem, but research has shown that it can boost your esteem by 40%.

· Assertive speech- Train yourself to speak without the filler words in your speech. Also, train your voice to come out as steady and low pitched. A combination of the two makes you confident and in return, makes you feel good about yourself.

· Break from social media- We mentioned before that social media is good, but it makes some of us compare our lives with others we think are doing better. This break should enable you to define your value on your terms.

· Smile- Smiling makes us feel good. You should smile even when you don't feel like it. Smiling brings happiness to you and the people around you, and happiness makes us feel good about ourselves.

Chapter 12: A Few Final Words

I want to end this book by saying a few final words about Reiki. I know when you are first starting out this can seem almost impossible but if you just give it a chance and preform the self-healing, you will be amazed at what you will experience.

You can clear the energy of a room or home by using Reiki as well. There are those who feel that their home is full of disturbances, these are often caused by a poltergeist which is caused from negative energy that is being suppressed by a person. Many people do not know what to do when these occur and they jump to the idea that their house is haunted. You can offer your services to friend and family that are having negative experiences in their homes. It is also a good idea to use Reiki to clean the energy when you are moving into a new home.

When you are in the middle of a Reiki session with a client, you may notice that as your hands pass over certain places on their body your hands become heavy. You need to focus a little more as you go through your session because this usually means that there is low energy flow in the area or even an energy blockage.

Salt will help contain negative energy. When you are preforming a Reiki session, place a bowl of salt at the foot of the receiver, as you sweep down their body with your hands you are pushing the negative energy into the bowl. Do this three to five times and when the session is over wash the salt down the drain getting all of the negative energy out of the area and away from the person and yourself.

Repeating mantras while you are preforming Reiki can help you keep random thoughts out of your mind. There are traditional mantras you can repeat or you can make something up of your own expressing what you want from the session. For instance: I take total healing energy into myself, or As total healing flows through me I allow it to work for its greater purpose.

Whatever the mantra is that you choose, you should repeat it throughout the entire session, helping you to focus all of your thoughts on the Reiki.

There are those who can reach the level of Reiki master in just a few days, it all depends on how open you are to the process and how much you focus on it. You will not become a master in a few days if you only do one 20 minute self-session and you should not feel discouraged if you are not able to heal others in just a few days. Remember it takes time to become great at anything. Those who master Reiki in a few days are called natural healers, they have been channeling Reiki energy their entire life. For the rest of us it can take some time to master.

Finally, you should not worry if you see variations in Reiki training. The way one person teaches will be completely different from the way another person teaches. One person may focus more on balancing the entire body whereas another person may be a medical healer and focus more on the physical body. It is best if you can have a few teachers whether it be online or in person so that you can see different variations of Reiki and choose the one that works for you.

I hope that you can use everything that you have learned in this book to become a master at Reiki. I also hope that this book has helped you to understand what Reiki really is and what it is not.

Chapter 13: Self-Attunement To Reiki

The ceremony you're about to follow for this attunement is very similar in theme to the one you would have experienced had you gone to a Reiki Master.

It is just as powerful - in fact probably more so.

The Reiki Master would have used intention and breath to attune you.

You're going to use intention and water.

Water? Yes water.

You see water is not just vital for life - it also has some very special properties, which are only now being understood by our scientists.

And one of these special properties lies in the ability of water to...

Accept, store and transfer information.

What kind of information?

Any information – in any form!

Water can accept, store and transfer to other systems, such as living systems, the information contained within...

☐☐☐☐☐☐☐☐☐☐☐☐☐Photographs
☐☐☐☐☐☐☐☐☐☐☐☐☐Thoughts
☐☐☐☐☐☐☐☐☐☐☐☐☐Spoken Words
☐☐☐☐☐☐☐☐☐☐☐☐☐Written Words
☐☐☐☐☐☐☐☐☐☐☐☐☐Sounds
☐☐☐☐☐☐☐☐☐☐☐☐☐Prayers
☐☐☐☐☐☐☐☐☐☐☐☐☐Pictures
☐☐☐☐☐☐☐☐☐☐☐☐☐Music
☐☐☐☐☐☐☐☐☐☐☐☐☐Singing
☐☐☐☐☐☐☐☐☐☐☐☐☐Chanting

Yes, we know it sounds incredible, even a bit far-fetched.

But once you've seen the photographic evidence you'll know it to be true. Water changes its molecular structure when any of the above are actively directed at it.

(Please read Messages from Water Vol. 1 & 2 by Dr Emoto for more in-depth information)

There are only a few people doing research in this area at present.

And most scientists, of course, debunk everything that has been discovered – but what's new there.

They've debunked almost everything at one time or another. Heck, they probably still can't admit that bumblebees can fly!

Water can and does carry the energetic impulses – the energetic information – of anything consciously and intentionally directed towards it.

Whole tracts of polluted water have been restored to a cleaner condition just by the action of a few people praying for that outcome.

Loving thoughts make the crystalline structure of water beautiful...

...hateful thoughts make it ugly.

Beautiful music creates beautiful structure - some of the modern stuff makes it hideous.

Water is us

We're over sixty five percent water by weight and our brains are almost eighty percent.

Is it any wonder we're so impressionable?

Yes, the magic of water is immense and you're about to experience it for yourself.

The following attunement ceremony uses water that has been consciously altered.

Consciously altered, by you, to carry the power of the attunement process deep within your body.

Every cell will then begin to resonate with this new information making you a very powerful Reiki Master.

So, like we say - you're going to use intention and water and, oh yes, a bit of sound and color too.

But first things first – read through the whole of this section on what to do a couple of times before doing anything else...

...gather together everything you'll need the day before you've decided to carry out your attunement.

Then follow the sequence as written.

Okay? Off we go.

First of all you will have to decide on where you are going to carry out the attunement process. It is quite important that you're not disturbed, so somewhere you can be by yourself is best.

There's no great esoteric reasoning behind why this should be so, by the way.

Nothing terrible will happen.

It's just that any interruption will serve to break your concentration, focus and intention, that's all.

So make all the necessary arrangements to keep yourself uninterrupted, ahead of time.

Next decide on whether you want to make the ceremony more personal to you by having some of your favorite, soothing music playing in the background.

If so get your player and music set up.

Would you like to have incense and or candles burning? Make sure you've got them all to hand if you do.

And don't forget the matches.

Now decide if you want to sit or kneel during the initiation. It makes no difference to the attunement itself. Your only concern should be about comfort and what feels best to you.

Okay then, that's the space prepared.

Just make sure it's comfortable and has a 'nice' feel.

And by that we mean whatever feels nice to you.

A table or small clear space on the floor will also be needed.

The next thing to do is gather together seven glass tumblers.

Now we say tumblers here, but it doesn't matter if they are tall glasses or short ones. It doesn't even matter if they don't all match.

What does matter is that they are all plain, uncolored and have no pictures, patterns or motifs on them.

You will now need some card or paper in these seven colors...

Red, orange, yellow, green, blue, purple and white.

From each sheet of paper cut out a circle which is going to fit under the base of each of your seven glasses.

Kinda like coaster size would be good.

Then cut a narrow label size strip from each sheet as well.

If you go to:

http://www.chikara-reiki-do.com/coasters

You can see, and download, everything you'll need (apart from the glasses, of course. And if you've got a color printer you'll be good to go.

Okay then.

You should now have seven coaster size circles – one of each color – and seven labels – one of each color.

On the red circle, using either a pen or pencil, draw out the Power Symbol. On the red label size piece of paper, write out the sacred name 'Cho-Ku-Rei' three times.

Sellotape this label to one of your tumblers.

Take the orange circle and draw out the Mental/Emotional Symbol on it. Write out the Sacred Name 'Sei-He-Ki' three times on the orange label, and stick it on a separate tumbler.

Getting the idea?

On the yellow circle draw the Distance Symbol and write out the sacred name 'Hon-Sha-Ze-Sho-Nen' on the yellow label.

Yes, you got it – stick the label on one of your tumblers.

The green circle should have the Tibetan Master Symbol drawn on it. The green label should have 'Dai-Ko-Mio' written out three times, and then stuck to a tumbler.

With the blue circle draw the Usui Master Symbol and write out Dai-Koo-Myo three times on the blue label.

Yup, stick the label to a tumbler.

On the purple circle: the Fire Serpent Symbol with Raku written three times on the label stuck to a tumbler.

On the last circle, the white circle, draw out all the symbols and write all six sacred names three times each onto the white label.

Stick this label onto the last tumbler.

So, what have we got now?

Seven different colored circles each with the appropriate symbol drawn on it. Seven clear glass tumblers separately labelled with the appropriate Sacred Name.

If that's what you've got sitting before you, we're in business.

Now on the evening of the day before you intend to carry out your Reiki Self-Attunement, pour some filtered or bottled mineral water into each of your tumblers.

There doesn't have to be a lot of water in each tumbler, three or four mouthfuls is enough.

Just make sure the water comes above the level of the writing on the label. So if you don't like to drink much water – although you really should be drinking at least two liters every day – make sure you stick the labels as low down as you can get them on the glass.

Place the red-labelled tumbler on the red circle, the orange-labelled tumbler on the orange circle, the yellow-labelled tumbler on the yellow circle, etc until each tumbler is sitting on its matching colored circle.

Incidentally, all these tumblers with the colored circles under them are placed on your table, or on the floor of the space you cleared.

Please forgive us if you think we've written out these instructions too simplistically.

We're really not trying to insult your intelligence.

It's just that, sometimes, written routines can be hard to follow, especially if you haven't had the benefit of a practical demonstration first.

There's a color picture of exactly how everything should look here:

http://www.chikara-reiki-do.com/coasters

Okay then.

These tumblers of water are going to remain on the colored circles over night, so they need to be covered.

A clean towel will do fine as it's only to keep dust and insects out.

In the morning, just prior to your self-attunement, arrange the tumblers – still on their coasters - directly in front of where you will be sitting or kneeling.

You'll need to be able to easily reach each one without having to get up.

And please arrange them in the following order...

If you are right handed place the red-labelled tumbler on the right hand side of your table or space.

Next to it on its immediate left will come the orange labelled one.

Next to that the yellow, then the green, the blue, purple and then lastly the white.

If you are left handed place the red tumbler on the left side of your table or space, then the orange one on its immediate right followed by the yellow, green, blue, purple and white.

The reason for this way of placing, as you have probably already guessed, is because you're going to drink the water in sequence.

And it just makes them a lot easier to pick up.

Let's begin the Self-Attunement ceremony

If you have chosen to have some pleasant music playing in the background, put it on. Similarly light the candles and/or incense.

Kneel or sit down in front of your tumblers of water and allow yourself to relax fully.

Close your eyes, take a few really deep breaths and let all your cares just drift away.

When you feel that you are ready, open your eyes...

...Pick up the first tumbler – the red labelled one – and holding it up in front of your face with both hands, chant the Sacred Name, Cho-Ku-Rei out loud, 3 times, directing your voice towards the tumbler.

Hold the glass for a few moments, and then drink the water. Do so intending and knowing that both the Symbol and the Sacred Name are being completely absorbed into your body, mind and spirit.

Put the tumbler to one side, pick up the second one – the orange labelled one – and repeat the process, chanting aloud, three times, the Sacred Name written on the glass.

Continue the process until you have chanted into, and drunk the water of, all seven tumblers.

Yes, with the seventh one you will have to chant the names of all six separate Sacred Names – three times each.

Now, gently close your eyes once again and just sit still for a few moments.

When you're ready...

Draw out, in the air just above your left palm, the Usui Master Symbol using the fire finger of your right hand.

Imagine that you are really drawing the Symbol onto your palm but without touching it.

Intend that the Symbol will sink into your palm just like butter does into hot toast. As you are doing this quietly, loudly or silently chant the Sacred Name Dai-Koo-Myo three times.

Now do exactly the same thing over the palm of your right hand using the fire finger of your left.

Bring both hands flat together at the front of your chest, as if praying, and hold them like this for a few moments, then return them to any comfortable position.

Raise your dominant hand (right hand if you're right handed, left if you're left handed) to a position over your crown.

Using your fire finger point directly down at the top of your head and draw out the Raku symbol.

Breathe in deeply and imagine the symbol being absorbed into you.

As you are doing this say out loud or silently to yourself...

"I open myself up to Divine Love and Wisdom".

Pause for a few moments and feel the symbol infusing your body.

Now draw out the Usui Master Symbol in the same place, breathe it in deeply and repeat...

"I open myself up to Divine Love and Wisdom".

Pause – as above.

Continue with this process using the Tibetan Master Symbol, the Distance Symbol, the Mental/Emotional Symbol and then finish with the Power Symbol.

Always breathe the Symbol deeply into yourself and whilst doing so say...

"I open myself up to Divine Love and Wisdom".

Always pause and feel the symbol infusing you.

Okay, nearly finished.

Using the same method as above draw the Raku Symbol in front of your third eye (a point roughly in the center of your forehead).

Breathe it in, and yes, repeat the phrase...

"I open myself up to Divine Love and Wisdom".

Draw out the Usui Master Symbol in front of your throat. Breathe it in whilst saying the phrase.

Next use the Tibetan Master Symbol in front of your heart center (a point on the midline of your body directly between your nipples). Breathe it in and say the phrase.

Now draw out the Distance Symbol in front of your solar plexus (a point on the midline of your body approximately 2 to 3 inches below the end of your breast bone). Breathe it in – say the phrase.

Draw out the Mental/Emotional Symbol in front of your Dan Tien (approximately 2 to 3 inches below your tummy button. Breathe it in – say the phrase.

Last one. Draw out the Power Symbol in front of your genital area. Breathe it in – say the phrase.

Sit for a few moments, then when you feel ready draw out a large Power Symbol in front of you – by large we mean the whole length of your body – breathe it into yourself and say...

"I seal this process with Divine Love and wisdom".

Okay – you're done. You are now a Reiki Master.

Not only are you a Usui Reiki Master, a Tibetan Reiki Master but also a Chikara-Reiki-Do Master too.

So...

CONGRATULATIONS

Well now, how do you feel?

If this is just your first read through and you haven't actually carried out the initiation ceremony yet - you've probably realized...

...how important it is that you can draw out the symbols, and say their Sacred Names, completely from memory...

...haven't you?

It just makes the job a whole lot easier. It flows better. It feels more powerful.

If you have carried out the attunement...

Welcome – Reiki Master – you make the world a better place simply by being here.

Now, if you'd prefer to be guided through this routine with Judith you may be interested in our Ultimate Reiki Package here:

http://www.chikara-reiki-do.com/master-kindle/

So, what's just happened?

Well, by leaving the tumblers on the colored circles over night the water absorbed and stored the...

• Reiki Symbols

• The Sacred Names

• The seven colors

As you drank the water the energetic information absorbed by the water, further enhanced with your chanting, was transferred to you.

Because the seven colors used are the same as those of the seven Major Chakras (the major energy centers of the body), each Sacred Symbol and Sacred Name was carried to, and absorbed into, the appropriate Chakra.

What does that mean?

It means that each energy center of your body is now 'attuned' to, and responds to, your intention to use Reiki energy.

Traditional Reiki Attunements only focus on the Crown, Third Eye and Palm Chakras. You have focused your intention on – thereby 'attuning' - all the Major Chakras, which means the whole of your body now resonates with the Reiki energy. (We've included a page giving more info – for those interested - at the end of the book).

Welcome then, to Chikara-Reiki-Do.

The 'whole body' Reiki.

Chapter 14: Mastering Reiki

You should always begin your Reiki practice by doing sessions on yourself. Once you are confident in healing yourself, if you have the desire to, you can also learn to heal the flow of energies through other people. It is generally advised once you are ready to advance your practice that you learn from a professional. However, this chapter will guide you through the basics.

Three Degrees of Reiki

Reiki practice is something that has different levels, with the lowest level being reserved for people who want to practice Reiki on themselves and the highest level is reserved for people to learn from and become Reiki masters.

First Degree Reiki

This involves self-care and constitutes of training that allows you to practice Reiki in daily life. Many people trained in First Degree Reiki can also place their hands on family and friends to promote Reiki healing. It is not uncommon for people in the healthcare field to learn First Degree Reiki, as it can be used as complementary medicine. Usually, massage therapists, nurses, and other people who are in a profession where it is appropriate to touch patients study First Degree Reiki.

Second Degree Reiki

Second Degree Reiki is practiced across a distance. It is ideal for situations where touch might not be possible or when it is inappropriate, such as in the case of psychotherapists who may want to learn Reiki to help patients to process emotional trauma. Second Degree Reiki relies on creating a mental connection, rather than a hands-on approach. In other situations, the mental connection may be established to enhance the effects of the Reiki session and promote a greater flow of energy.

Third Degree Reiki

Third Degree Reiki is the highest level, being achieved only by Reiki masters. To officially earn certification as a Reiki master, it is generally accepted that you must receive an invitation from an existing Reiki master. The people who are extended this invitation are those who have devoted their lives to the practice of Reiki and teaching it to others. Since it requires an invitation from a Reiki master, Third Degree Reiki is generally learned through a long apprenticeship.

Reiki Attunement

A major component of practicing Reiki is the vibrational frequency. You can only channel the healing energies of the Universe that you have been attuned to. It is not uncommon for a Reiki attunement to be performed before someone moves up to the next degree of Reiki since increasing your vibrational frequency will allow you to increase your healing potential.

A Reiki attunement can be done by a Reiki teacher who possesses the ability to open your chakras in a way that allows a higher state of consciousness to flow through you. To be able to make your energy flow through someone else, these chakras must be able to put forth and absorb energy, connecting you to the flow of life energy in the universe and allowing you to channel it through someone else's body. The process of Reiki attunement may also be called expanding your energy channels. If you do not want to work with a Reiki teacher, then you may also be able to raise your vibrational frequency by doing Chi exercises, which were discussed in the Chakras chapter.

Additional Therapies

Often, Reiki is not used as a standalone therapy. While it can produce results on its own, especially when it is performed by someone who has earned the title of Reiki Master, there are additional therapies that can be used to increase the results of Reiki healing. This section will go over some of them so that you can get the most of your Reiki healing sessions.

Crystal Therapy

Crystals are made up of elements of the earth. They carry unique vibrational energy depending on what they are made out of. This vibrational energy allows them to attune to your body, producing certain effects. It is not uncommon for people to wear certain stones or carry them around. They can also be used during Reiki and other practices, as a way to enhance the results.

To add crystals to your Reiki session, you can put your hands into position over the chakras as you focus your intention and your healing energy. Hold the appropriate crystal in your hand and channel the energy into yourself or the person you are healing. The crystal that you use depends on which chakra you are trying to heal, excite, or calm. You can choose whichever crystal has the strongest pull or seems to call to you, or you can choose one that goes with the specific chakra you are trying to heal. Here are some of the crystals that should be used for each of the chakras:

- Crown Chakra- Clear Quartz, Diamond, Ametrine, Clear Calcite, Amethyst/ Violet
- Third Eye Chakra- Lazuli, Lapis/ Indigo, Quartz, Sodalite
- Throat Chakra- Turquoise/ Blue, Celestite, Blue Lace Agate, Aquamarine
- Heart Chakra- Pink Calcite, Emerald/ Green, Rose Quartz, Tourmaline
- Solar Plexus Chakra- Amber/ Yellow, Malachite, Aragonite, Moonstone, Topaz
- Sacral Chakra- Carnelian, Orange Stones, Smoky Quartz, Red Jasper
- Root Chakra- Lodestone/ Red, Bloodstone, Tiger's Eye, Ruby, Garnet, Hematite

Something to keep in mind is that crystals can take on negative energy as people would. Some people choose to release negative energy on their crystal by performing a Reiki session to clean the crystal's aura before their own. There are several other options, including burning sage to cleanse the crystal or soaking it in saltwater. Some people also bury their crystals in salt, especially if they are soft and will be harmed by a saltwater bath. To amplify the power of a crystal, you can stick it on a windowsill or in direct moonlight. This works best when the moon is highly visible.

Pray or Meditate

Many people stay away from the prayer option because they believe they must claim a religion or choose a specific God if they are to pray. However, prayer does not have to be directed at anyone or anything specific. If you are not comfortable praying, you could also meditate.

This is a time when you should focus on your intentions. Get in the habit of focusing on the positives of what you want. Instead of saying that you do not want pain, say that you want to heal. Even when you say something negatively, by reflecting on it as you meditate, you are giving it your focus and energy. This can draw that thing into your life or cancel out what you are trying to achieve with the prayer.

You should always look at meditation and prayer as an opportunity to reflect and look inward. Even if you are speaking outward, whether to your God, the Universe, or whatever you believe in, it is important to look inward. Speaking out loud can help trigger insights that you may not have realized otherwise.

It does not matter how long you pray or when you pray. Set aside time each day, whether a few minutes or longer. Make it a habit. If you can, speak out loud as you pray and focus on the things that you need to be happy in your life.

Yoga

Yoga originally comes from India. However, it has recently become popular around the world. It is used for physical activity but also encourages the development of a more spiritual mindset.

The type of yoga that you participate in has a lot to do with the effects, as the positions and breathing patterns can invoke certain results.

As you do yoga, you should always use the breathing practice called 'Pranayama.' It is all about concentrating on your breathing to clear your mind of all unnecessary thoughts. Also, it helps make you feel calm and relaxed. A simple breathing exercise you can follow is find a quiet place and you can either sit or stand according to your convenience. Take a deep breath through your nose (count to four), hold your breath (count to four), and exhale through your mouth (to the count of four), and wait (to the count of four). You can repeat this until you feel calm and relaxed. This type of breathing is necessary for people who are trying to bring results to their yoga session. It allows you to connect with the Universe, while improving your physical and mental strength, increasing your memory power, and even extending your lifespan. You can take a class for yoga. Alternatively, look up positions or videos online. You'd be surprised how much information is available once you know where to look!

Serve Others

We may do the things that our family, friends, and co-workers ask us regularly. However, fewer people take time out of their busy weeks to help those who truly need it. The reality is that every person is fighting a battle that nobody else understands. For example, someone homeless is not necessarily lazy— they are the result of a collection of life circumstances that could just as easily happen to you or me.

As you start to explore the world and help the people that truly need it, you will find yourself better prepared to help others. You will find a newfound sense of satisfaction in yourself and the responsibilities of life, as you realize that you can be responsible for more than just your normal day-to-day routine. As a person that connects to the Universe, you have the knowledge and wisdom to help those around you. Additionally, helping those who are less fortunate allows you to gain your maturity, strength, and knowledge when it comes to fighting battles in your life.

Nourish Your Soul

Nourishing the soul is all about learning those things that make you happy and bring you peace— and then making an effort to do them. When you work long hours or have a hectic family life, it is hard to find time for yourself. It is important to remember that you owe yourself this nourishment. It is necessary for you to take care of yourself if you want to connect to the Universal consciousness and connect with others.

In addition to nourishing yourself by committing time to yourself, it is essential that you take care of your physical body and mind. Be sure that you get enough sleep each night. Practice relaxation techniques if you need to. You should also choose nutrient-dense foods, rather than those that are filled with empty calories. By nourishing your body and mind, you will find yourself in the best possible state to encourage mental, emotional, and spiritual healing and wellness too.

Be Mindful in Your Experience

People lead busy lives. As you rush from task to task, when do you make time to slow down? Think back to the last time that you had a meal. Were you rushing to get back to whatever task you were doing before or even checking your emails while you ate? What about your last trip to the store or work? Did you look around you as you went and observe the sights, or were you on autopilot mode as you just tried to get from A to B?

It is easy to become so immersed with the physical experience that we forget to slow down and experience the world in all its beauty. Instead of going on autopilot, make an effort to notice the things you are doing. When you are washing dishes or sweeping the floor, pay attention to the way the muscles move in your arms, shoulders, and back. As you eat, pay attention to the different flavors and textures you are getting from the food. Immerse yourself in the experience of eating and chew slowly enough that you can take it all in. Whenever you are driving or walking, notice your surroundings. Instead of staring at the carpet when you are rushing to your office in the morning, make an effort to smile at your coworkers. It doesn't take any extra time to move the muscles in your face. By immersing yourself in your human experience, you will find yourself more connected to your spiritual one as well.

Chapter 15: How And Where To Apply Reiki

The Application Room
Where and how should we give and receive a Reiki session?
Reiki is love!
Reiki is harmony!
Harmony is beauty!
So, let's take maximum care of the place where we are going to act and be organized: love, harmony, and beauty. The environments collect energies; they are left with feelings and thoughts on file. Sometimes, there may have been fights and discussions in the environment. These harmful energies remain archived in the place, being able to harm the treatment of Reiki.

To perform Reiki treatments, the ideal would be an environment reserved exclusively for this purpose in order to avoid these harmful vibrations and energies. In the event that this environment is not available, it is essential that the Reikian make an energy cleaning treatment in the environment before.

Level I Reikians, who are not yet fit for the use of ambient cleaning symbols, can use the following mental technique. A violet light that flows and cleans the entire environment is first visualized, then a white light to energize it, and later, a golden light to seal the environment against negative vibrations coming from outside.

Once this procedure is done, any room can be used for Reiki. The recommendations to follow are for those who wish to work with Reiki professionally. The place must be very clean and always well-painted with white or light colors, giving preference to green and blue. We must avoid any other exciting colors, such as red or yellow.

It is important that you have at least one window to ensure good ventilation in order to reduce harmful positive ions. Natural floors, especially wood and synthetic ones (eucatex, carpets, etc.), should be avoided, and if the floor is made of cement, marble, or granite, carpets and pillows made of natural fibers may be placed on them.

It is convenient to limit the number of paintings and ornaments on the walls that are a source of distraction. Depending on the size of the enclosure, put enough live plants that, in addition to decorating, help keep the room energetically clean. The luminosity should be discrete and indirect, being advisable to use a switch to regulate the intensity of the light. Too much light is stressful.

Soft and relaxing music is very important, both to create a suitable atmosphere, and to create an energetic complement (sound therapy) for the treatment. There is very nice music specially composed to practice Reiki, in which the minutes provided for each position are cadenced within the music itself as very soft, reminder signs. If you don't have it, use soft and relaxing music that must be chosen carefully, for example, Gregorian chants, bird sounds, flowing water, wind sounds, etc. The new era and classic, if you like them both, use incense (air element). Those of oriental manufacture are excellent and cheap. It is not only about perfuming the environment, making it more pleasant, but also favoring the reception of energy. Instead of the incense, we can use aromatic diffusers, which are small glass or ceramic containers where water and natural essences are placed in the upper part. Place a small candle in the lower part. Energetically, it is important to always keep a burning candle (fire element), whatever it is, during the development of the work.

A glass of water (water element) is recommended. And we must change it between one session and another.

A crystal or an amethyst (earth element) can be used near the patient; it will radiate transmutation energy.

It is important a container with coarse salt (NaCl), which must be replaced periodically. The (NaCl) (sodium chlorate) transmutes the negative vibrations or remains of the patient's emotions that would remain in the environment. The comfort of the practitioner and the patient is essential, advising the use of a hammock or healing table with the appropriate height so that the Reikiano can sit or stand during the session. The use of a clean cotton handkerchief under the cast patient is appropriate and should always be changed between sessions. The treatment can last an hour or more, and if you do not have a specific table, you can substitute a dining or work table, with a foam mat or cover.

The soil is the least suitable place to administer cures due to the telluric energies that remain impregnated on the floor, but, in an emergency, if it were the only place available, use it.

How to Proceed With Your Application to Other People

The color of the therapist's clothes does not matter. It must be comfortable and clean to avoid negative energy impregnations in widely used clothes. Reiki energy passes smoothly through clothing and other materials, so it is not necessary for the patient to remove it.

All metal ornaments, both from the receiver and the practitioner, rings, bracelets, chains, crystals, and watches must be removed. These have their own vibrations that can interfere with Reiki energy. A medal, a ring, or a bracelet that cannot be removed for religious reasons will not cause great interference.

Therapists who use stones in healing processes know that they should be cleaned regularly, and, if they were not purified, they would not be able to heal, or worse, they "will be sick." Stones saturated with negative energy radiate equivalent emanations. That also applies to metals, glasses, and plastics. The jewels used daily come into contact, permanently, with all kinds of energy vibration, and are usually saturated with ambient energy. We observe people whose headaches disappear when they begin to wash their eyes regularly with running water. Then, trying to create an atmosphere as free as possible from any interference, remove all jewels before applying Reiki.

To avoid the absorption of etheric waste, before starting the application, we must wash our hands with running water. We will do the same at the end to break the auric interaction. If, for some reason, water is not available, we will obtain the same energy cleaning effect by exposing our hands to the flame of a candle for a few moments. We must ensure that we are not interrupted by the arrival of another person or by a phone call.

If desired, the therapist can say a silent prayer in gratitude for the grace of being able to act with divine energy and function as a bridge and channel of universal energy. Under no circumstances should we insist that people receive Reiki. It is optional for everyone to wish to improve.

We must do the centralization of the heart always and in any type of treatment, taking into account that all the energy that will enter through the coronary chakra will pass through the cardiac chakra, which, if harmonized, makes the person a better channel. The Reikian should not be emotionally involved with the patient's problem or create expectations regarding the results. The receiver must be reminded that he does not need to think about anything, in particular, that energy will flow freely, and that one can also speak during the session. The flow of Reiki energy is not interrupted. However, silence is ideal.

Before starting the application, smooth the patient's aura in order to establish the first contact. You can repeat this

162

procedure three times. This ritual serves to establish the first contact with the patient and to balance the aura. It is as if "before knocking on the door," instead of entering without announcing.

Reiki is a method of balancing the totality of being; the disease is a visible fragment of an unbalanced system and will be healed from the moment. A state of harmony is reached. This process of harmonization, triggered by Reiki energy, will be completed in the time designated by the higher consciousness of the person being treated. In general, it will take four to twenty-one sessions to heal 80 percent of the problems you encounter. However, remember that Master Takata, in 1936, had a tumor and needed four months of daily application to recover at Dr. Hayashi's clinic in Tokyo. Therefore, do not raise expectations about the duration of treatment.

You are a Reiki channel; what heals is the energy of God, so remember that the honor belongs to him. Sincere Reikiano does not allow himself to be venerated or worshiped because of healing. Because it is only one channel, it will not be responsible in case of healing, often due to lack of continuity in treatment and lack of mental hygiene. Also, karmic factors may play a part.

Avoid making diagnoses, such as medical prerogative. It does not interfere with the treatment the other person is undergoing. Remember that Reiki is an alternative and also complementary therapy. Consequently, use it as a complementary therapy.

The quantity and quality of Reiki in the application are determined by the recipient. Therefore, act cautiously against creating reaction patterns and stimuli. Sometimes, people may feel heat, tingling, palpitations, and vibrations. Many times, they may feel nothing or just a slight relaxation; feeling or not feeling is not a parameter to judge the efficiency of the treatment.

It is not uncommon to be in tune with the patient's discomfort. Normally, the recording of discomfort in the Reikian occurs in the same part of the body where the patient's pain is located. However, that does not mean that the facilitator has or will remain with the symptom of the recipient. That fact occurs because, during application in another person, you will be participating in a common auric field.

If those feelings were unpleasant, it is enough that we change position or interrupt the application for a few seconds. Those feelings are not residual. In the event that unpleasant sensations persist, analyze the reasons for being in vibrational tuning with that state and check your self-treatment, intensifying it. When starting any treatment, especially in serious diseases, it is advisable to make three applications in a row, for three consecutive days, thus facilitating a faster response of the immune system, but that is not a rule. The therapist and the other person must jointly establish the schedule of applications, according to the time availability of both.

Try to find out the reasons for the situation that led the person to be willing to receive Reiki. Such a procedure helps and facilitates a safe course for the application, and we can choose the most specific positions for the case.

Both the patient and the therapist must keep legs, fingers, and arms without crossing them so that all the energy channels of the body can receive the same amount and remain equally unlocked and clean. Throughout the session, the practitioner should seek a comfortable position, support the back, relax the shoulders, and if possible, support the arms.

The application time in each position at level I is five minutes, while the complete treatment takes seventy minutes since they are fourteen basic positions. But there is no impediment to dedicate a shorter time of application, and even not to do all the positions. To choose some, follow your intuition. Sensitize yourself to the energy field of the other person and feel what is most appropriate to each situation. The ideal is the complete treatment. However, if it becomes impossible, little Reiki is better than none.

As for the hands, the Reikian will keep the fingers together and the shell-shaped hand, slightly curved so that there is no dispersion of energy as if we were drinking water, although without stressing them and leaving them flexible and soft.

The treatment should begin with the head, following all conventional positions, with the hands gently placed. Position changes, whenever possible, are made by moving just one hand at a time, so as not to interrupt contact. To apply energy to the genital region, it is convenient to use a folded towel or blanket over that part of the body to avoid misunderstandings. Another way is to place the suspended hands, two or three centimeters from the body, or ask the receiver to place their hands on the area. Then, we will apply energy through the patient's hands.

After the treatment, it is advisable, being at the therapist's discretion, to thank God, in silent prayer, for the opportunity to have been able to work for someone as a Divine channel. In order to break the interaction of auric fields, the therapist should wash their hands with running water after finishing the session. Or rub your hands vigorously and blow toward them to cut off contact with the person treated, causing the flow of Reiki to cease, or, ultimately, use a flame.

The payment of therapies is lawful, necessary, and correct, within the full respect of the law of nature that requires the free exchange of energy. The Reikian charges for the time spent as a channel in the treatment, and not for the Reiki energy, which is divine, gifted, and unlimited.

After treatment, it is common for both to feel a sense of peace, intense relaxation, and deep sleep, let the patient rest a certain period of time later. It is recommended, after the change of the handkerchief, of the water and, if necessary, of the salt, of the candle, of the music and of the incense, that the therapist rests for at least fifteen minutes, between one session and another. The ideal thing to do would be meditating. Reiki can also be applied to animals, seeds, and plants.

Chapter 16: What Is Reiki And How Does It Work?

Imagine if you were able to heal yourself, as well as your loved ones, with the help of the energy that surrounds you? Wouldn't that be terrific?

Everything around us, including ourselves, is made of, and is full of energy. With this fact in mind, I have two pieces of good news that I would like to share with you:

The energy that surrounds us is unlimited. We do not run out of it.

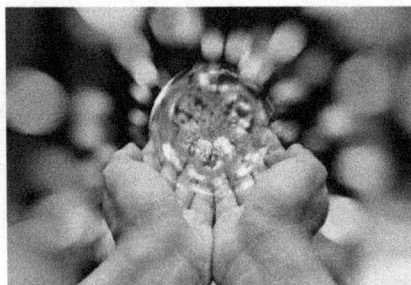

You don't have to use your own "reserves" of energy to power yourself or fuel your endeavors. You can learn to take that energy from your surroundings, and effectively utilize it to help yourself and/or the people around you.

Sounds amazing, right? Maybe even a little grandiose?

Well, what if I told you after reading this book, you will be able to do just exactly that—to harness the energy of your surroundings in order to benefit both you and the ones you love. Sounds like a great concept, right? Honestly, it's less of a theory and more of a practical system; one that you will now learn.

Reiki 101

You have most probably heard of Reiki before. At the same time, you probably don't know what it is exactly (which might well be one of the reasons you bought this book).

The word **Reiki** comes from Japanese origin. The word **Ray** means 'spirit,' or 'soul'. And the word **Ki** translates to 'energy,' or 'mind'.

Reiki is a healing system, one that views all human illnesses and diseases from the point of view of energy. The basis of Reiki is built around the methodology that energy — excessive or a lack of — within human organs, is the foundational basis for health or disease.

If distortion of the energy shell (body) of a person is detected, a Reiki master saturates this zone with his/her own life energy - "*ki*". This energy that the master uses is synthesized by him from the surrounding space (cosmos). This, in turn, creates a channel of pure energy of Reiki, one which feeds the damaged organs and systems of the patient, restoring all distortions in their energy shell. This way, the body is being healed in totality, not just locally. Consequently, health is restored and all the body functions are normalized and stabilized, restoring the patient in question to a state of homeostasis.

Unlike conventional energy healing where the healer usually works with his own energy (including using his kundalini energy), Reiki masters use the "pure" energy of space, which is easily absorbed by a person. And precisely because it is pure, and not tainted by the healers own energy, the energy that is drawn and used from our universal surroundings is much more potent in its healing abilities.

Nowadays, there are many different courses, seminars, centers, Reiki schools, training systems, and directions founded by various Reiki masters. One of the most famous versions is Kundalini Reiki, which is based on the activation of Kundalini energy in the human body and its subsequent use to heal your physical body, mind, and to help other people.

There are also different other types of Reiki, such as Mikao Usui Reiki and Karuna Reiki, which are named after the master teachers who founded these Reiki schools and whose systems are divided into certain levels, where students receive the appropriate initiations and ranks (1st Reiki level, 2nd Reiki level, 3rd Reiki level).

This book will teach you how to use the energy within you and around you, and how to help yourself and your loved ones too.

It will help you find harmony within the inner and outer world, and will lead you to a happier, healthier, and more fulfilled life.

How Does Reiki Work?

Before we begin, please take a look at the list below. If any of the 'symptoms' seem familiar, it means that you could likely use some Reiki in your life.

9 Signs That Your Soul Needs Reiki

You feel like you're 'lost', have reached a dead end, and cannot find your way out of a situation

Sometimes you feel like a failure and/or a loser. Everything you touch seems to fall apart

You seek support, understanding, and acceptance, but you can't seem to find it, not even from your loved ones

From time to time, everything seems meaningless and you feel like quitting and giving up on everything

There's always an annoying bustle in your life, a never-ending list of things that need to be done. This leaves you feeling like you have absolutely no time for yourself

You're tired. You can barely get up in the morning. You feel like you have no strength, no energy, no ideas, and no inspiration

You have an urge to heal yourself, to seek an escape from everything, or to spend time alone with yourself, to listen to the sound of silence, and hear the whisper of your soul

With all the spiritual practices and the knowledge you have acquired, all of them seem to fall short of helping you cope with situations in your life

You are experiencing bouts of obsession, anxiety, fear, or you feel let down all the time

Do any of these symptoms feel familiar? If so, then you are definitely on the right track by reading this book.

Another good thing is that Reiki therapy helps you connect with your soul and find a way out of practically any situation in your life. And it does so without the need for you to fall out of the rhythm of life you're used to, or requiring you to hide in Himalayan caves for years.

Reiki is an affordable and relatively straightforward method by which to significantly improve your overall wellbeing and condition on both a physical and mental level. The practice helps you to find harmony within yourself and establish positive contact with the world around you — affording you the opportunity to realize what the meaning of life is.

The Mystery of Reiki

Reiki practice has a very deep history. To be succinct, the system was traditionally used for healing in ancient Japan.

Although healing is still the main focus and purpose of the system, Reiki in the modern world is still surrounded by the controversial (and often disputed) question: "Is Reiki a sect?"

Arguments over this issue have persisted for many years. And, since the attitude towards this practice is rather ambiguous, the theories surrounding the origins and purpose of the system has spread like a wildfire of gossip and conjecture.

An example of one of these doubt-inducing practices is the fact that people who have undergone Reiki initiations go on to hold regular gatherings, and the master who performed the original ritual ascends to the role of spiritual mentor of the recipient.

Many people say that Reiki is a sect because the seminars necessarily include talks about the merits of Mikao Usui, the founder of Reiki. His photo is placed on an altar, in front of which various rituals are held.

There are many organizations that seek to earn a lot of money by promoting Reiki, promising miraculous healings from various ailments, including cancer. Because of this, many people have grown to view Reiki as a sect.

However, the practices of Reiki can be done on their own too, allowing you to gain all the benefits of the system, and doing so completely free of charge.

Reiki Philosophy

The doctrine of Reiki is practiced in all corners of the Earth, and every year the number of people who join the practice increases.

Depending on the person's abilities and the duration of their practice, three main levels of Reiki exist. And each time, there is an initiation process held. At each step, new opportunities are opened up to the practitioner of Reiki.

Stage 1: The first stage practices and teaches mastery of what is known as 'The Laying of Hands'. At this stage, the practitioner is taught how to lay their hands in a way that can transfer and concentrate the energy in your body, into living beings.

Stage 2: At the second stage, the practitioner studies the symbols of Reiki and learns to work with the past and the future. At this stage, the practitioner begins to learn how to utilize the energy of the Universe in order to impact emotional and physical change. This stage is where the practitioner begins to unlock the power within the Reiki system and methodology.

Stage 3: At the third stage, the practitioner is considered a Master, and they are now free to teach and conduct initiations.

Reiki Psychology

The modern world constantly keeps us in a state of flux. We seem to always be chasing something. Whether it be financial goals, well-being, comfort or other benefits, we can get tangled in the chase and forget about the important things that are really needed for happiness and a sense of inner harmony.

By studying the beautiful art of Reiki and learning how to apply what you learn from the system, you gradually free yourself from the invisible shackles that modern-day life seems to routinely imprison people with.

We gain this freedom by becoming realigned with what our true values are, and remembering the true selves that we lost touch with during the 'rat race' of day-to-day life.

The meditations found within Reiki also helps you to isolate yourself from any problems — bringing you perspective — and allowing you to find yourself and the beat of your inner peace.

Regular practice of Reiki gives you a chance to get rid of psychological problems too, setting you free from your emotional calluses, and ultimately allowing you to change your life for the better.

Reiki Esoterism

There are many different techniques that a person can use in order to heal their body or soul or even change their destiny.

Within Reiki, there are certain symbols that allow the practitioner to harness the energy that surrounds us all (we will be covering these in more detail later in the book).

The symbols attune the practitioner to various types of Universal energies, and when connected with the human body these energies provoke powerful reactions, ones that can be used for healing or self-development.

An example of this in practice can be found in the following powerful technique: Fill a glass with water, look at it, and then visualize a selected Reiki symbol. Do this meditation for a total of 120 seconds

After focusing on the Reiki symbol for the allotted time, switch your focus to a goal or desire that you wish to come true. Do this for 60 seconds

This will charge the water with Reiki energy.

Drink the charged water in small sips, while imaging the realization of your wish.

Reiki is a Journey

Anyone can learn Reiki practices, but you need to be aware that it will take time and effort to develop the necessary knowledge and skills.

Conclusion

The next step is to take what you have learned within this book and apply it to your own life so that you, too, may experience everything that we discussed. Learning about Reiki is only one step of the process, but education alone is not enough to actually reap any of the benefits that are possible. Instead, you must utilize it in your life and experience the healing for yourself so that you can lead a more healthy and productive life.

If you have never had a Reiki session done before, now is the time to look around and find a practitioner in your area. It is impossible to truly understand what you learned unless you undergo a session for yourself. As we discussed, it is unique and tailored to each individual client. Make sure that you take your time when finding someone to heal you though, as not every client-healer pairing is going to be the right one. If possible, talk to the practitioner before you book and see if their energy is a match for you. This entire experience is meant to help you, so never feel bad about passing on someone who simply does not feel right. Reiki sessions can get expensive, and you don't want to feel like you wasted your time or money on someone who didn't help you in any way.

Maybe through reading this book, you felt inspired, and the topics that were discussed stirred something in you that you cannot explain. Many times, people are drawn to the topic of Reiki because they have a calling in this area, and the fact that you picked up a copy of this book could be an indication that it is something you should explore further. Becoming a healer is a beautiful process, one that will transform your life and give you purpose and meaning. You can make a real impact on the lives of others by practicing this art, and if you feel drawn to that path, then make sure you pursue it.

Find a Reiki school can all be done online, and there are many all across the globe. Listen to your own gut and intuition, and do not deny yourself a new experience if that is what you are interested in. Having goals, motivation, and striving towards something bigger than ourselves is all a part of what Reiki is, and as both a practitioner and as a client, we are participating in making the world a slightly better place. The more positive energy that flows from us and into our environment, the more people we can have an impact on and change. We have the ability to do this. It just comes down to learning how that is possible

CPSIA information can be obtained
at www.ICGtesting.com
Printed in the USA
BVHW071041060820
585686BV00010B/726

9 781989 990308